Guide to the
Code of Ethics
for Nurses

Interpretation
AND
Application

EDITOR: **Martha D. M. Fowler**, PhD, MDiv, MS, RN, FAAN

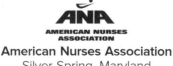
AMERICAN NURSES ASSOCIATION
American Nurses Association
Silver Spring, Maryland
2010

nurses books.org

Library of Congress Cataloging-in-Publication data
Guide to the code of ethics for nurses : interpretation and application / Marsha D.M. Fowler, editor.
    p. ; cm.
    Includes bibliographical references and index.
    ISBN-13: 978-1-55810-258-3 (pbk.)
    ISBN-10: 1-55810-258-2 (pbk.)
    1. Nursing ethics. I. Fowler, Marsha Diane Mary. II. American Nurses Association.
    [DNLM: 1. Ethics, Nursing--Guideline. 2. Codes of Ethics--Guideline. 3. Societies, Nursing--
        Guideline. WY 85 G946 2008]
    RT85.G85   2008
    174.2--dc22   2008004469

The American Nurses Association (ANA) is a national professional association. This ANA publication—*Guide to the Code of Nursing: Interpretation and Application*—reflects the thinking of the nursing profession on various issues and should be reviewed in conjunction with state board of nursing policies and practices. State law, rules, and regulations govern the practice of nursing; *Guide to the Code of Nursing: Interpretation and Application* guides nurses in the application of their professional skills and responsibilities. The opinions in this book reflect those of the authors and do not necessarily reflect positions or policies of the American Nurses Association. Furthermore, the information in this book should not be construed as legal or professional advice.

Published by Nursesbooks.org
The Publishing Program of ANA
www.Nursesbooks.org

American Nurses Association
8515 Georgia Avenue, Suite 400
Silver Spring, MD 20910-3492
1-800-274-4ANA
www.Nursingworld.org

The American Nurses Association (ANA) is the only full-service professional organization representing the interests of the nation's 3.1 million registered nurses through its constituent member nurses associations, its organizational affiliates, and the Center for American Nurses. The ANA advances the nursing profession by fostering high standards of nursing practice, promoting the rights of nurses in the workplace, projecting a positive and realistic view of nursing, and by lobbying the Congress and regulatory agencies on health care issues affecting nurses and the public.

DEVELOPMENT EDITOR: Rosanne O'Connor Roe (ANA staff)
PRODUCTION EDITOR: Eric Wurzbacher (ANA staff)
COPYEDITING AND INDEXING: Grammarians, Inc., Alexandria, VA
DESIGN & COMPOSITION 2010: David Fox, AURAS Design, Silver Spring, MD
PRINTING: McArdle Printing, Upper Marlboro, MD

ISBN-13: 978-1-55810-258-3   SAN: 851-3481   30M   07/10R

First printing February 2008. Second printing July 2008. Third printing February 2009.
Fourth printing (with new cover) July 2010.*

*This book was re-issued with a new cover in July 2010. All content other than the annotations on this page and on page 137 is identical to that which was first published in February 2008 and subsequent reprints. (See page 137 for guidelines on citing the content of Appendix A.)

Contents

Acknowledgments

The American Nurses Association would like to thank the following people for their help in reviewing the content of this book:

Laurie A. Badzek, JD, LLM, MS, RN, NAP
Janet M. Dahm, PsyD, RNC
Barbara J. Daly, PhD, RN, FAAN
Anne J. Davis, PhD, DS, MS, RN, FAAN
Candia B. Laughlin, MS, RN-BC
Kathleen M. Poi, MS, RN, CNAA
Molly Sullivan, MAOL, RN
Carol R. Taylor, PhD, MSN, RN
Linda S. Warino, BSN, RN, CPAN

Permissions

The American Nurses Association gratefully acknowledges the publishers' permission to reproduce passages from the following publications.

Chapter 5

Burgess, Mary Ayers. 1928. The hospital and the nursing supply. *Transaction of the American Hospital Association*, pp. 440–414. Chicago: AHA.

Jameton, Andrew. Duties to Self: Professional Nursing in the Critical Care Unit, in Fowler, Marsha and Levine-Ariff, June (eds.). *Ethics at the Bedside*. Philadelphia: JB Lippincott, 1985, pp. 115–135.

Chapter 8

Cooper, R. W., G L Frank, C A Gouty, and M M Hansen. 2003. Ethical helps and challenges faced by nurse leaders in the healthcare industry. *Journal of Nursing Administration* 33(1): 17–23.

DeVries, R., and J. Subedi, eds. 1998. *Bioethics and Society: Constructing the Ethical Enterprise*. Upper Saddle River, NJ: Prentice Hall, p xiii.

Lee, M. B., and I. Saeed. 2001. Oppression and horizontal violence: The case of nurses in Pakistan. Nursing Forum 36(1): 15–24.

Oberle, K., and S. Tenove. 2000. Ethical issues in public health nursing. *Nursing Ethics* 7:425–38.

Page–Sikma, S. K., and H. M. Young, 2003. Nurse delegation in Washington state: A case study of concurrent policy implementation and evaluation. *Policy, Politics, & Nursing Practice* 4(1): 53-61.

Shapiro, H. T. 1999. Reflections on the interface of bioethics, public policy, and science. *Kennedy Institute of Ethics Journal* 9(3): 209–24.

Weston, A. 2002. *A Practical Companion to Ethics*, 2nd ed. New York: Oxford University Press., p 12.

Chapter 9

Perlman, C. H., Olbrechts-Tyteca, L. *The New Rhetoric: A Treatise on Argumentation*. Notre Dame: Notre Dame University; 1969. p. 51.

Winter, Gibson. *Elements for a Social Ethics*. NY: Macmillan; 1966, p. 215.

About the Authors

Provision 1

Carol R. Taylor, PhD, MSN, RN, is a faculty member of the Georgetown University School of Nursing and Health Studies and Director of the Georgetown University Center for Clinical Bioethics. She is a graduate of Holy Family University (BSN), the Catholic University of America (MSN), and Georgetown University (PhD in philosophy with a concentration in bioethics). Bioethics has been a focus of her teaching and research since 1980 linked to her passion to "make health care work" for those who need it. Special interests include healthcare decision making and professional ethics.

Provision 2

Anne J. Davis, PhD, DS, MS, RN, FAAN, and Professor Emerita, taught at the University of California for 34 years. Beginning in 1962, Dr. Davis's career focused on international work with appointments in Israel, India, Nigeria, Ghana, Kenya, Japan, Korea, China, and Taiwan. These rich experiences led to the development of her overriding interest in cultural diversity and nursing ethics. She is a graduate of Emory University in Atlanta (BS, Nursing), Boston University (MS, Psychiatry), and University of California, Berkeley (PhD, Higher Education). Dr. Davis has been the recipient of numerous awards, including an honorary Doctor of Science from Emory University and election as a Fellow in the American Academy of Nursing.

Provision 3

John G. Twomey, PhD, PNP, is an Associate Professor at the Graduate Program in Nursing at the MGH Institute of Health Professions in Boston, Massachusetts. Dr. Twomey's doctoral work was in bioethics. He teaches bioethics and research and serves on several human subjects research protection committees. He has completed two National Institute of Nursing Research-supported post-doctoral fellowships in genetics. A member of the International Society of Nurses in Genetics, he does research in the area of the ethics of genetic testing of children. He is the editor of the Ethics Column in the Society's quarterly newsletter.

Provision 4

Laurie A. Badzek, JD, LLM, MS, RN, NAP, is currently Director of the American Nurses Association Center of Ethics and Human Rights, a role in which she previously served from 1998–99. During that time, Badzek was instrumental in developing a plan that ultimately resulted in the approval of a new Code of Ethics for Nurses by the 2001 House of Delegates. Currently a tenured, full professor at the West Virginia University School of Nursing, Badzek, a nurse attorney, teaches nursing, ethics, law, and health policy. Having practiced in a variety of nursing and law positions, she is an active researcher, investigating ethical and legal healthcare issues. Her current research interests include patient and family decision making, nutraceutical use, mature minors, genomics, and professional healthcare ethics. Her research has been published in nursing, medical, and communication studies journals, including *Journal of Nursing Law, Nephrology Nursing Journal, Annals of Internal Medicine, Journal of Palliative Care,* and *Health Communication.*

Provision 5

Marsha D.M. Fowler, PhD, MDiv, MS, RN, FAAN, is Senior Fellow and Professor of Ethics, Spirituality, and Faith Integration at Azusa Pacific University. She is a graduate of Kaiser Foundation School of Nursing (diploma), University of California at San Francisco (BS, MS), Fuller Theological Seminary (MDiv), and the University of Southern California (PhD). She has engaged in teaching and research in bioethics and spirituality since 1974. Her research interests are in the history and development of nursing ethics and the Code of Ethics for Nurses, social ethics and professions, suffering, the intersections of spirituality and ethics, and religious ethics in nursing. Dr. Fowler is also a Fellow in the American Academy of Nursing.

Provision 6

Linda L. Olson, PhD, RN, CNAA, is currently Professor and Dean of the School of Nursing at North Park University in Chicago, Illinois. Previously, she taught courses in healthcare policy and economics, leadership, and nursing service administration at the graduate and undergraduate levels as an Associate Professor at St. Xavier University in Chicago. She has prior experience in nursing service administration, practice, and consultation. Dr. Olson received her PhD and MBA from the University of Illinois at Chicago, and her baccalaureate and master's degrees in nursing from Northern Illinois University. Her area of research interest is the work environment, particularly focusing on organizational culture and ethics. As part of her dissertation work, she developed the research instrument, the Hospital Ethical Climate Survey, which has also been used by several researchers, nurses, and others in the United States and internationally. She was a member of the ANA Task Force to Revise the Code of Ethics, as well as the Congress on Nursing Practice and Economics, and has held numerous leadership positions at local, state, and national levels. In addition, she serves as an appraiser for the Magnet Recognition Program.

Provision 7

Theresa S. Drought, PhD, RN, is currently an Assistant Professor at the University of Virginia School of Nursing. She has long been interested in the ethical issues related to professionalism in health care, serving as a nurse consultant to the California Medical Association's Council on Ethical Affairs, chair of the ANA\C Ethics Committee (ANA/California), and as a member of the American Nurses Association Task Force that produced the 2001 Code of Ethics for Nurses. Her publications and research address issues of professionalism and ethics in nursing and end-of-life decision making. Her current research focuses on decisions made by stranger surrogates. She received her PhD in nursing from the University of California at San Francisco in 2000.

Elizabeth G. Epstein, PhD, RN, received her PhD in Nursing from the University of Virginia in 2007. In August 2007, she took a position as Assistant Professor at the University of Virginia School of Nursing. Her doctoral dissertation and continuing interests are in ethics and end-of-life issues in the pediatric setting. In particular, she is interested in studying moral distress and moral obligations among healthcare providers, as well as determining how care-based ethics is evident in pediatric end-of-life care. She is a member of the American Society for Bioethics and Humanities. She serves as a facilitator for Conversations in Clinical Ethics, a multidisciplinary group at the University of Virginia that meets to discuss ethical issues that arise in the hospital setting.

Provision 8

Mary C. Silva, PhD, RN, FAAN, received her BSN and MS from the Ohio State University and her PhD from the University of Maryland. In addition, she undertook postdoctoral studies at Georgetown University. She has taught healthcare ethics at the master's and doctoral levels and published extensively in the area of ethics, beginning in the 1970s. She is currently Professor Emerita at George Mason University in Fairfax, Virginia. Dr. Silva is also a Fellow in the American Academy of Nursing.

Provision 9

Marsha D.M. Fowler, PhD, MDiv, MS, RN, FAAN, is Senior Fellow and Professor of Ethics, Spirituality, and Faith Integration at Azusa Pacific University. She is a graduate of Kaiser Foundation School of Nursing (diploma), University of California at San Francisco (BS, MS), Fuller Theological Seminary (MDiv), and the University of Southern California (PhD). She has engaged in teaching and research in bioethics and spirituality since 1974. Her research interests are in the history and development of nursing ethics and the Code of Ethics for Nurses, social ethics and professions, suffering, the intersections of spirituality and ethics, and religious ethics in nursing. Dr. Fowler is also a Fellow in the American Academy of Nursing.

Preface

A code of ethics stands as a central and necessary mark of a profession. It functions as a general guide for the profession's members and as a social contract with the public that it serves. The group that would eventually become the American Nurses Association first discussed a code of ethics in 1896. When the ANA code of ethics was first developed, it was used as a model by nursing organizations elsewhere in the world, so it had considerable influence both in this country and internationally. As American nursing education and practice advanced over the years since then, and we developed a deeper understanding and appreciation of ourselves as professionals, the code has been updated on several occasions to reflect these changes. However, the core value of service to others has remained consistent throughout. One major change that can be found is the re-conceptualization of the patient. Formerly limited to an individual person usually in the hospital, now the concept of the patient includes individuals, their families, and the communities in which they reside. Another change of great significance, detailed in the fifth provision of the code, reminds us that nurses owe the same duties to self as to others. Such duties include professional growth, maintenance of competence, preservation of wholeness of character, and personal integrity. Just as the health system and professional organizations need to attend to the rights of patients, they also must support nurses and help them to take the actions necessary to fulfill these duties.

You will need to read this Code carefully and repeatedly to reflect on these nine provisions for what they mean in your daily life as a nurse. Ethics and ethical codes are not just nice ideas that some distant committee dreamed up. Rather, they are what give voice to who we as professional nurses are at our very core. This Code reflects our fundamental values and ideals as individual nurses and as a member of a professional group.

When the ANA House of Delegates first unanimously accepted the Code for Professional Nurses in 1950, years of consideration had been given to the development of this code, consideration that continues to this day. The ANA modified the Code in 1956, 1960, 1968, 1976, 1985, and 2001 so that it could continue to guide nurses in increasingly more complex roles and functions. These revisions reflect not only the changing roles and functions of nurses and their relationships with colleagues, but also and, more important, the commitment of professional nursing to maintaining one of its most important and vital document that continues to inform nurses, other health professionals, and the general public of nursing's central values. These values underpin this Code of Ethics. Read it often and use it wisely.

And finally, join me in thanking the latest ANA task force for their excellent work in revising our Code.

Anne J. Davis, PhD, DS, MS, RN, FAAN
Professor Emerita, University of California, San Francisco
Professor, Nagano College of Nursing, Japan
Former Chair, ANA Ethics Committee

Introduction

The Code Of Ethics For Nurses: Something Old And Something New

The American Nurses Association's (ANA) *Code of Ethics for Nurses with Interpretive Statements* (ANA, 2001) was never intended to be carved in stone for all eternity. Rather, it was meant to be a document that has naturally evolved and developed in accord with the changing social context of nursing, and with the progress and aspirations of the profession. However, despite the changes over time in the Code's expression, interpretation, and application, the central ethical values, duties and commitments of nursing have remained stable. The Code of Ethics for Nurses is the profession's public expression of those values, duties, and commitments. An understanding of the conventional history of this document and its various revisions over time is prerequisite to understanding the current Code of Ethics for Nurses.

The first generally accepted code of ethics for nursing in the United States was written in 1893 by Lystra Gretter, principal of the Farrand Training School for Nurses, in Detroit, in the form of a pledge patterned after medicine's Hippocratic Oath. Gretter felt that Florence Nightingale embodied the highest ideals of nursing and, consequently, named the first version of the Code the "Florence Nightingale Pledge." The Nightingale Pledge was generally accepted in this country in its original version, and was usually administered at school of nursing graduation exercises, even after ANA adopted its first official code of ethics in 1950. The Nightingale Pledge reads as follows:

> I solemnly pledge myself before God and in the presence of this assembly: To pass my life in purity and to practice my profession faithfully. I will abstain from whatever is deleterious and mischievous, and will not take or knowingly administer any harmful drug. I will do all in my power to elevate the standard of my profession, and will hold in confidence all personal matters committed to my keeping, and all family affairs coming to my knowledge in the practice of my profession. With loyalty will I endeavor to aid the physician in his work and devote myself to the welfare of those committed to my care (Gretter, 1910).

The original Nightingale Pledge has served as the basis for numerous Hollywood portrayals of nurses, and it continues to be administered at nursing school graduations to this day. In 1896, three years after the appearance of the Nightingale Pledge, the delegates and representatives of the Nurses' Associated Alumnae of the United States and Canada (renamed the American Nurses Association in the early 1900s) met at the Manhattan Beach Hotel in New York to establish their constitution and articles of incorporation. The first purpose of the group was "to establish and maintain a code of ethics" (Minutes, 1896). However, despite the recognized significance of a code of ethics for the profession, 54 years were to lapse before a Code was officially adopted.

In 1926, A Suggested Code was provisionally adopted by ANA and published in the *American Journal of Nursing (AJN)* [ANA, Committee on Ethics, 1926]. Critical comments were sought from the *AJN* readership. The first proposed Code was written in the flowery narrative style characteristic of the late 1800s and early 1900s. Although somewhat idealized, it was a solid document, admirably unwavering and professionally astute in its statement of the values of the profession at the time. However, despite its rhetorical elegance, it did not enumerate specific principles at a more practical level as the membership had hoped, and so the Suggested Code was not adopted.

In 1940, A Suggested Code was replaced by A Tentative Code, also published in *AJN* (ANA, Committee on Ethics, 1940). This 1940 version of the Code incorporated verbatim some sections from the Suggested Code. Both codes were organized around the theme of categories of relationships, such as nurse-to-profession or nurse-to-patient. The emphasis of the 1940 Code, however; demonstrated a more overt concern for the status and public recognition of nursing as a profession. As with the 1926 Suggested Code, comments were sought from *AJN* readers.

Subsequent debate, inquiries, and expressions of concern formed the basis for an entirely rewritten version in 1949. The revised Tentative Code was submitted to ANA members, professional groups, schools of nursing, and healthcare agencies for comment. In addition, input was solicited through the use of a questionnaire mailed to groups and individuals, resulting in 4,759 responses (Flanagan, 1976). *The Code for Professional Nurses* was unanimously accepted by the ANA House of Delegates in 1950 (ANA, 1950). At last, the profession had an official code of ethics! The style of the 1950 Code differed dramatically from that of the two previous, unadopted versions. It consisted of a brief preamble and 17 succinct, enumerated provisions. This Code relinquished the overt use of professional relationships as its organizing framework.

It did, however, incorporate many elements of relationships within its provisions. Following adoption of the 1950 Code, debates were held and comments were periodically sought from *AJN* readers. Responses from readers and others formed the basis for a minor emendation to the Code, made in 1956. A 1950 provision, which proscribed advertising, was revised at this time. This provision originally read:

> Professional nurses do not permit their names to be used in connection with testimonials in the advertisement of products. (ANA, 1950).

The provision was revised to read:

> Professional nurses assist in disseminating scientific knowledge through any form of public announcement not intended to endorse or promote a commercial product or service. Professional nurses or groups of nurses who advertise professional services do so in conformity with the standards of the nursing profession.

Apart from that small change, the first *major* revision of the 1950 Code was developed in 1960 (ANA, 1960).

Between 1950 and 1960, attention shifted from concern for the content of the Code to concern about its enforcement in the practice setting. Subsequent changes in the ANA bylaws incorporated provisions relating to the obligations of association members to uphold the Code. Thus, in 1964, the ANA Committee on Ethics developed the *Suggested Guidelines for Handling Alleged Violations of the Code for Professional Nurses* (ANA, 1964).

The next major revision of the Code was formally adopted in 1968. This revision dropped the term "professional" from the title to indicate that the Code applied to both technical and professional nurses. The 1968 revision also omitted the preamble of the 1960 Code, and condensed the number of provisions from 17 to 10 (ANA, 1968). Although the 1968 revision shortened the number of provisions, it still carried forward all the concerns of the 1960 Code, incorporating them either implicitly or explicitly. However, an important omission in the 1968 Code pertained to the personal ethics of the nurse. The 1968 Code was the first version to omit references to the "private ethics" of the nurse, and the demand that the nurse "adhere to standards of personal ethics which reflect credit upon the profession" (ANA, 1950). The personal sphere was no longer deemed to fall within the purview of professional scrutiny. Given the early focus of nursing educators and administrators on questions of the moral purity of the probationer, trainee, and graduate, this is both a significant and substantive change. Additionally, the 1968 Code was the first version that did not explicitly mention the physician; "members of other health professions" are mentioned, but the physician is not singled out (ANA, 1968). During the 1970s, significant changes in nursing and its social context made another revision to the Code necessary.

In 1976, a new version of the Code was formally adopted. Among other changes, this version of the Code created a new emphasis on the responsibility of the patient to participate in his or her own care. The notions of nursing autonomy and the nurse-as-advocate were addressed as well. The 1976 Code also shifted to a predominant (though not consistent) use of the term *client* rather than *patient*, and a consistent use of nonsexist terminology (ANA, 1976).The 1985 revision of the Code retained the provisions of the 1976 version, yet included revised interpretive statements. In some cases, these new interpretive statements significantly clarified, redirected, or altered the sense of the original provisions. For instance, the 1976 interpretive statement for provision 11 declared that "quality health care is mandated as a right to all citizens" (ANA, 1976). The 1985 interpretive statement made citizenship irrelevant to any consideration of access to or distribution of nursing or healthcare services (ANA, 1985).

In 1995, a Task Force for the Revision of the Code for Nurses was convened to evaluate the need for a revision of the Code. The Task Force determined that not only did the interpretive statements need revision, but the Provisions themselves, unchanged for 23 years, also needed revision. The Task Force identified a number of concerns that needed to be addressed in a new revision. These included a need to expand the Code's reflections of approaches to ethics that would include virtue and feminist, communitarian, and social ethics. The committee wished to see an enlarged concern for global health; for the conditions that produce disease, illness, and trauma; and for nurse participation in health policy. Economic constraints that could result in a workplace environment that posed a risk to patients or nurses needed increased attention. In addition, the Task Force wanted the Code to encompass all nurses, in all positions, in all venues, and the work of professional nursing associations. In some places, certain moral language needed clarification, such as "refusal to participate," which needed to incorporate a discussion of "conscientious objection" as a moral ground for "refusal to participate."

The Task Force was also concerned with reuniting "personal" and "professional" ethics and heightening recognition that the nurse has duties to self. The Task Force undertook this thorough revision of the Provisions as well as the interpretive statements with an acute awareness of the tradition of nursing ethics and a commitment to retaining our moral identity from the past and continuing to bring it into the present. This revision of the Code was faced with a different process of approval from previous Codes. In the reorganization of the structure of ANA, the new Code and its interpretive statements would go before the House of Delegates for approval. Previous codes required approval of the House for the provisions, but not for the interpretive statements.

The interpretive statements had previously been subject to revision and approval by the Committee on Ethics alone. However, in the reorganization, the Committee on Ethics was dissolved. The new revision of the Code's provisions and interpretive statements was formally adopted by the ANA House of Delegates in 2001. The Code of Ethics for Nurses must of necessity undergo periodic revision in order to remain relevant. However, the Code is framed in such a way as to address categories of concern, rather than specific events or changes in the workplace. This is done to keep the Code "elastic" so that it need not be changed with every wind that blows. The Code might mention "natural disasters" and discuss a nurse's responsibilities in such disasters, but it would not mention specific earthquakes, hurricanes, or tsunamis. The Code will address nursing "in clinical settings," but will not mention specific settings such as intensive care units, retail nursing, or parish nursing. In that way, the Code would not need revision every time a new venue for nursing arose. The Code will address treatments or interventions generically, or categories of treatment such as "the administration of food and fluid," but will no longer specify specific treatments lest the code need to be revised every time a new treatment is developed. In general, it is understood that the broader provisions of a Code will require revision substantially less frequently than will the more specific interpretive statements.

To date, these have been the successive revisions of the Code:

1893—Florence Nightingale Pledge (informal standard)

1926—A Suggested Code (unadopted)

1940—A Tentative Code (unadopted)

1950—Code for Professional Nurses

1956—Code for Professional Nurses, amended

1960—Code for Professional Nurses, revised

1968—Code for Professional Nurses, revised

1976—*Code for Nurses with Interpretive Statements*

1985—*Code for Nurses with Interpretive Statements*, revised

2001—*Code of Ethics for Nurses with Interpretive Statements*

Though these versions of the Code vary in their articulation of the duties and values of the profession, they also contain important features that remain relatively unchanged. For instance, while nurses always were urged not to discriminate on the basis of creed, nationality, or race (ANA, Committee on Ethics, 1940), contemporary nursing has broadened that concern to disallow discrimination on the basis of any personal attribute, socioeconomic status, or nature of the health problem itself (ANA, 1976). The 1985 Code claims that "all national, ethnic, racial, religious, cultural, political, educational, economic, developmental, personality, role, and sexual differences" are unjust grounds for discriminating among those in need of care (ANA, 1985).

The 2001 Code is even more emphatic: "The need for health care is universal, transcending all individual differences. The nurse establishes relationships and delivers nursing services with respect for human needs and values, and without prejudice" (ANA, 2001). The primary ethical principle of justice remains a central concern; it is the expression of that principle that has developed over the successive revisions of the Code. Within the Code for Nurses, whatever the version, there is a deep and truly abiding concern for the social justice at every level; for the amelioration of the conditions that are the causes of disease, illness, and trauma; for the recognition of the worth and dignity of all with whom the nurse comes into contact; for the provision of high-quality nursing care in accord with the standards and ideals of the profession; and for just treatment of the nurse. These are consistent and historic concerns of the profession that have been reflected, more strongly at some times than at others, in the successive revisions of the Code. The "new Code" reflects the "old Code" in its continuity with nursing's moral past; thus, the 2001 Code is a shiny, new, genuine antique.

The Code for Nurses reflects both constancy and change—constancy in the identification of the ethical virtues, values, ideals, and norms of the profession, and change in relation to both the interpretation of those virtues, values, ideals, and norms, and the growth of the profession itself. It is comforting to note that the moral duties and values of the profession were set in place long before the dizzying and sometimes chaotic forces of contemporary science and technology added to the burdens of clinical decision making. Though no easy task, ethical decision making in the nursing profession is not adrift—it is firmly anchored to the distinguished, distinctive, and definitive moral and ethical tradition of the nursing profession as represented in the Code of Ethics for Nurses. As you read each of the chapters that follow, you will see in them nursing's moral past, present, and future.

Marsha D.M. Fowler
Professor of Ethics
Spirituality and Faith Integration and Senior Fellow
Institute for Faith Integration
Azusa Pacific University
Azusa, CA

Associate Pastor
First Congregational Church of Los Angeles
Los Angeles, California

References

American Nurses Association. 1950. *ANA House of Delegates Proceedings*, Vol. I. New York: ANA.

American Nurses Association. 1960. *ANA House of Delegates Proceedings*. New York: ANA.

American Nurses Association Committee on Ethics. 1964. *Suggested Guidelines For Handling Alleged Violations of the Code for Professional Nurses*. New York: ANA.

American Nurses Association. 1968. *ANA House of Delegates Reports*, 1966–1968. New York: ANA.

American Nurses Association. 1976. *The Code for Nurses with Interpretive Statements*. Kansas City, MO: ANA.

American Nurses Association. 1985. *The Code for Nurses with Interpretive Statements*, revised. Kansas City, MO: American Nurses Publishing.

American Nurses Association. 2001. *The Code of Ethics for Nurses with Interpretive Statements*. Washington, DC: Nursesbooks.org.

American Nurses Association Committee on Ethics. 1926. A Suggested Code. *American Journal of Nursing* 26(8): 599–601.

American Nurses Association Committee on Ethics. 1940. A Tentative Code for the nursing profession. *American Journal of Nursing* 40(9): 977–980.

Flanagan, L. 1976. *One Strong Voice.* Kansas City, MO: ANA.

Gretter, L. 1910. Florence Nightingale Pledge: Autograph manuscript dated 1893. *American Journal of Nursing* 10(4): 271.

Provision One

The nurse, in all professional relationships, practices with compassion and respect for the inherent dignity, worth, and uniqueness of every individual, unrestricted by considerations of social or economic status, personal attributes, or the nature of health problems.

Provision One

Carol R. Taylor, PhD, MSN, RN

History of this Commitment

The Nightingale Pledge, which is patterned after medicine's Hippocratic oath, is generally accepted as the first nursing code of ethics. While it contains a pledge that the nurse devote herself to the welfare of those committed to her care, it does not explicitly mention compassion and respect for human dignity. Similarly, the earliest code drafted by the American Nurses Association in 1926 mentions only devotion. A Tentative Code, published in *The American Journal of Nursing* in 1940 but never adopted, contains the following statements:

> The nurse should carry out professional commitments and activities with meticulous care, with a generous measure of performance, and with fidelity toward those whom she serves. Honesty, understanding, gentleness, and patience should characterize all of the acts of the nurse. A sense of the fitness of things is particularly important (ANA, 1940; p. 978).

> The nurse has a basic concern for people as human beings, confidence in the fundamental power of personality for good, respect for religious beliefs of others, and a philosophy which will sustain and inspire others as well as herself (ANA, 1940; p. 980).

In the 1950 Code for Professional Nurses, a substantive revision of A Tentative Code, we find for the first time:

> Need for nursing service is universal. Professional nursing service is therefore unrestricted by considerations of nationality, race, creed or color (ANA, 1950; p. 110).

This statement became the first provision of the 1968 Code for Professional Nurses:

> The nurse provides services with respect for the dignity of man, unrestricted by considerations of nationality, race, creed, color or status (ANA, 1968).

In 1976, the Code added the following important content to this provision:

The nurse provides services with respect for human dignity *and the uniqueness of the client* unrestricted by considerations of *social or economic status, personal attributes, or the nature of health problems* (emphasis added) (ANA, 1976; p. 3).

In addition to signaling the uniqueness of each recipient of nursing care (then newly termed "the client"), the 1976 Code also recognized that things other than nationality, race, creed, color, and status can result in unacceptable differences in treatment. This provision remained the same in the 1985 Code. In the 2001 revision, the scope was broadened to include "all professional relationships" so that "respect" is now broadened to include "*inherent* dignity (a critical modifier), *worth*, and uniqueness." A significant addition was the phrase "*practices with compassion* and respect." The addition of the virtue compassion was related to the serious scholarship currently being done by nurse ethicists in virtue theory and care ethics. Also noteworthy was the replacement of the term client with "every individual," so that the Code now states that:

The nurse, *in all professional relationships, practices with compassion* and respect for the *inherent* dignity, *worth*, and uniqueness of every individual, unrestricted by considerations of social or economic status, personal attributes, or the nature of health problems (emphasis added) (ANA, 2001).

It is important to recognize that the drafters of the Code of Ethics for Nurses have continued to identify respect for persons as a core ethical principal, including respect for autonomy in this principle (Interpretive Statement 1.4, Right to Self-determination). Although *The Belmont Report* (National Commission for Behavioral Research, 1979) identified respect for persons, beneficence and justice as the three basic ethical principles, Beauchamp and Childress in their *Principles of Biomedical Ethics*, now in its fifth edition (2001), popularized four principles of biomedical ethics: autonomy, beneficence, nonmaleficence, and justice.

As bioethics in the United States evolved, autonomy replaced respect for persons in most lists of core principles. While the emphasis on autonomy was understandable in a country struggling to correct the abuses of paternalistic medicine, its narrower focus ignores bigger challenges related to inherent dignity and worth. Strikingly absent from popularized versions of the principles of bioethics is responsiveness to human vulnerability. The Code of Ethics recognizes the many factors that result in injustices in health care and holds nurses to a high standard of compassion and respect for all—especially those most vulnerable. As recent national studies continue to prove, great disparities in health outcomes in the United States continue—making Provision 1 an ideal not yet realized (AHRQ, 2006).

Nurse ethicist Barbara Jacobs recommends respect for, or the restoration of, human dignity, as a common central phenomenon to unite and reflect nursing theory and practice (Jacobs, 2001). *Consilience*, a way to unify the knowledge that is needed to support this phenomenon, is suggested as one example of a possible approach toward a philosophy of nursing that embraces multiple forms and sources of knowledge in all-encompassing morality that ultimately ennobles the lives of all human beings in covenantal relationships with nurses both in theory and in practice.

Thinking Beyond This Provision

Most nurses will tell you that they entered nursing to "help others," and few at first will admit to being biased or discriminatory in their professional relations. Honest reflection, however, results in most of us realizing that we respond to patients and other professional caregivers differently based on numerous factors, not the least of which are race and ethnicity, age, financial status, position/title, body size, health, and other personal attributes. We probably all think of those with whom we interact professionally as falling into one of three categories: people for whom we'd do anything—even at great personal cost; people whom we give their due; and people we serve grudgingly, if at all. It is to be hoped that few nurses can identify individuals with whom they interact professionally who fall into a fourth category: people they aim to harm by disrespectful behavior or worse.

To the extent that we admit to some degree of difference in our ways of relating to others, Provision 1 presents us with a challenging ideal:

> The nurse, *in all professional relationships*, practices with compassion and respect for the inherent dignity, worth, and uniqueness of every individual, unrestricted by considerations of social or economic status, personal attributes, or the nature of health problems (emphasis added).

Provision 1 is not claiming that every nurse needs to have "warm and fuzzy" feelings for all encountered professionally—that would be unrealistic. Certain patients, members of their families, and even other healthcare professionals, will fill us with frustration, anger, sometimes even disgust and revulsion, but the Code mandates that we have a professional obligation to move beyond these feelings and, at the very least, to recognize the humanity of others and respond with compassion and respect. At times, this can be a heroic effort and may even require the support of the professional caregiving team.

It is helpful for nurses to be reflective concerning the fundamental assumptions about people they bring to practice. Reflect on the following statements and check those with which you agree. Compare your list with that of a colleague and explore any differences. Talk about the consequences of the assumptions you hold for yourself, your patients, your colleagues, and the public at large. Which of your assumptions are consistent with Provision 1 of the Code of Ethics? How should colleagues respond to individuals with convictions that violate Provision 1 of the Code of Ethics?

- Every human being, merely by virtue of being human, merits my equal and full respect.

- The more vulnerable people are because of illness, frailty, or other marginalizing factors, the *more* they command my compassion and respect.

- The more vulnerable people are because of illness, frailty, or other marginalizing factors, the *less* they command my compassion and respect.

- I agree that I need to be compassionate and respectful to those innocently affected by disease, injury, or frailty—so long as self-abusive behaviors did not cause the disease or infirmity

- People need to earn my respect.

- It is only human and ethically justifiable to respect people differently.

Interpretive Statement 1.4, the right to self-determination, mandates that nurses be knowledgeable about the moral and legal rights of all patients to be self-determining. Many critics of contemporary health care bemoan the failure of all healthcare professionals, including nurses, to promote patients' authentic autonomy. Respect for autonomy in many cases is now reduced to not interfering with a patient's expressed choices. This is a far cry from what nurse ethicist Sally Gadow initially described as existential advocacy:

> The ideal which existential advocacy expresses is...that individuals be assisted by nursing to authentically exercise their freedom of self-determination. [A] uthentic... [means] a way of reaching decisions...truly one's own—decisions that express all...one believes important about oneself and the world. ... (Gadow, 1980; p. 85).

How many nurses today know their patients well enough to facilitate authentic autonomy? And how many nurses value existential advocacy such that they are willing to fight for institutional cultures that demand nothing less.

Applying the Provision: Rethinking Professional Relationships and What has Historically Been Termed "The Therapeutic Use of Self"

In every human encounter, we convey one of three messages: (1) *Go away, my world would be better without you;* (2) *You are an object, a task to be done, you mean nothing to me;* or (3) *You are a person of worth, I care about you.* The more vulnerable people are, the more we can become their world of meaning. Since disease, injury, and illness can separate people from affirming experiences that enhance their sense of worth (family relationships, work, other achievements), how we present ourselves as health professionals to individuals needing care truly matters. A quick moment of reflection will help you to identify individuals in your own life whom you perceive as being either therapeutic or toxic presences. How do you think your patients and colleagues would evaluate your presence? What do you leave in your wake: affirmation, peace, joy, warmth, support, the experience of being cared about as well cared for? In healthcare settings, it is critical for nurses to relate to patients as a healing presence. Two stories follow to illustrate this point.

A friend of mine named Laurie, who has cancer, wrote to me after a visit to an infusion therapy center:

> The nurse came into my room and touched me on the forearm. It wasn't a furtive nurse searching for a vein thing. It wasn't "I'm a nurse, you're a patient, too bad" thing. It was "I'm a human being, you're a human being, how are you?" thing. *And that one touch rendered tolerable everything else she had to do that morning.*

Powerfully illustrated in this example are the profound consequences of human touch and compassionate, respectful presence. Contrast this illustration with the next.

Another friend diagnosed with advanced ovarian cancer spent two long, hard years dying. She was president of our college, had a PhD in biology, was from Worcester, Massachusetts, and had that delightful New England sense of reserve and privacy. She was one of the most gentle, loving human beings I have ever had the blessing to know. She had intestinal obstructions and was in and out of the hospital constantly. I remember spending hours simply sitting behind her to lend physical support as she retched over an emesis basin. She instructed me to tell my students the following:

Guide to the Code of Ethics for Nurses

When I first got sick, it didn't matter how people treated me because I knew who I was. But now that I've grown weaker I become whomever people make me. If a nurse walks into my room and moves me like meat, I become meat!

It made me want to cry that I or a member of my profession had the capacity to take a Lillian and transform her to a slab of meat by virtue of how I gazed, what I said or failed to say, or how I touched. This is the power that is ours. At the end of the shift, have people been left better or worse for having experienced us?

Reflect on the following case studies in light of Provision 1 of the Code of Ethics.

Case Example 1

Jean Thatcher is a morbidly obese, 47-year-old, single, white attorney with multiple sclerosis. She is frequently admitted to your hospital for complications related to her multiple sclerosis and obesity. Since she quickly "exhausts" the patience and best efforts of the staff, she is "rotated" among several units all of whom know her well and loathe her inpatient stays on their unit. The staff's best efforts to educate her about appropriate self-care and preventive practices have fallen on deaf ears. She refuses to cooperate when her support is elicited for bathing, position changes, and the like. Her one visitor, her mother, believes that the staff discriminates again her daughter and complains frequently to management. Both the patient and her mother frequently threaten to sue the hospital for neglect and discrimination. Jean admits that she is refusing to eat or help with bathing and positioning. She said she has "had enough" and wants to give up. Most of the staff have already "given up" and ask "why we should we try to help Jean when she has been clear about not wanting our help?" Today, one nurse was overheard saying, "I'm not going to sprain my back trying to get her to move when she refuses to cooperate. She can lie in her filth for all I care." The nurse manager calls a meeting to explore how the team can best respond to the challenges of caring for Ms. Thatcher. In what practical ways does Provision 1 of the Code of Ethics influence the standard of care for Ms. Thatcher and similar patients? Is Ms. Thatcher's wish to "give up" an autonomous act of self-determination that should be supported by her nurses? ■

Case Example 2

Mr. Rivera staggers into the emergency room at 2:00 a.m. complaining of belly pain. He speaks Spanish only. Well known to the ER staff, Mr. Rivera is homeless and has a history of alcoholism and violence. He has been blacklisted at several of the local shelters for homeless men. The night is cold and there is freezing rain. The resident called to examine Mr. Rivera does not "work-up" the complaint of "belly pain," instead saying that, once again, Mr. Rivera only wants a warm bed for the night, a bath, something to eat and meds to make him "feel good." The E.R. nurse manager instructs a nursing student to "clean up" Mr. Rivera when the day shift arrives. The nursing student finds him combative when aroused and asks for help only to be told to "do the best she can." His stools are dark and she suspects blood in the stool, but is told only to babysit the patient until he is discharged. In what practical ways does Provision 1 of the Code of Ethics for Nurses influence the standard of care for Mr. Rivera and similar patients? Does Mr. Rivera's previous history justify the lack of care he is receiving this admission? Is it justified to expect the nursing student to meet his needs unaided? How should the student's clinical instructor respond to the student when she complains about the staff's lack of compassion, professionalism, and aid? ■

Case Example 3

You are the director of nursing in a large nursing home. Your units are staffed primarily with licensed practical nurses and nursing assistants. Recently several nursing assistants have come to you complaining about unequal treatment in assignments and privileges. You know that there are some racial tensions among the staff, which is predominantly persons of African American and Hispanic identity, and suspect that these may be contributing to the conflict. While the nursing home allegedly has a "zero tolerance" policy for discrimination, you know that this is not always the case. What guidance does Provision 1 of the Code of Ethics offer to promote respectful professional relationships among the staff and residents? ■

References

All online references were accessed in December 2007.

Agency for Healthcare Research and Quality (AHRQ). 2006. *National Healthcare Disparities Report. 2006.* Rockville, MD: AHRQ. http://www.ahrq.gov/qual/nhdr06/nhdr06.htm.

American Nurses Association. 1926. A Suggested Code: A code of ethics presented for the consideration of the American Nurses' Association. *American Journal of Nursing* 26(8): 599–601.

American Nurses Association. 1940. A Tentative Code for the nursing profession. *American Journal of Nursing* 40(9): 977–80.

American Nurses Association. 1950. Code for professional nurses. *ANA House of Delegates Proceedings,* Vol. 1; New York: ANA.

American Nurses Association. 1968. Code for professional nurses, Revised. *ANA House of Delegates Proceedings,* Vol. 1; New York: ANA.

American Nurses Association. 1976. *Code for Nurses with Interpretive Statements.* Kansas City, MO: American Nurses Publishing.

American Nurses Association. 1985. *Code for Nurses with Interpretive Statements,* Revised. Washington, DC: American Nurses Publishing.

American Nurses Association. 2001. *Code of Ethics for Nurses with Interpretive Statements.* Washington, DC: American Nurses Publishing.

Beauchamp, T.L. and J.F. Childress. 2001. *Principles of Biomedical Ethics,* 5th ed. New York: Oxford University Press.

Cooper, L.A., and N.R. Powe. 2004. *Disparities in Patient Experiences, Health Care Processes, and Outcomes: The Role of Patient-Provider Racial, Ethnic, and Language Concordance.* New York: The Commonwealth Fund.

Gadow, S. 1980. Existential advocacy: Philosophical dimensions of nursing practice. In *Nursing Images and Ideals,* S. Spicker and S. Gadow, eds. NY: Springer Publishing Company.

Jacobs, B. 2001. Respect for human dignity: A central phenomenon to philosophically unite nursing theory and practice through consilience of knowledge. *Advances in Nursing Science* 24(1): 17–35.

Kaiser Health Disparities Report: A Weekly Look at Race, Ethnicity and Health. http://www.kaisernetwork.org/Daily_reports/rep_disparities.cfm

National Commission for the Protection of Human Subjects of Biomedical and Behavioral Research. 1979. *The Belmont Report: Ethical Principles and Guidelines for the Protection of Human Subjects of Research.* Washington, DC: U. S. Government Printing Office.

Smedley, B.D., A.Y. Stith, and A.R. Nelson, Eds. 2002. *Unequal Treatment: Confronting Racial and Ethnic Disparities in Health Care.* Washington, DC: National Academies Press.

About the Author

Carol R. Taylor, PhD, MSN, RN, is a faculty member of the Georgetown University School of Nursing and Health Studies and Director of the Georgetown University Center for Clinical Bioethics. She is a graduate of Holy Family University (BSN), the Catholic University of America (MSN), and Georgetown University (PhD in philosophy with a concentration in bioethics). Bioethics has been a focus of her teaching and research since 1980 linked to her passion to "make health care work" for those who need it. Special interests include healthcare decision making and professional ethics.

Provision Two

The nurse's primary commitment is to the patient, whether an individual, family, group, or community.

Provision Two

Anne J. Davis, PhD, DS, MS, RN, FAAN

History of this Commitment

From the beginning of professional nursing in the 1870s in the United States, after the Civil War when nurses served in military hospitals, nursing care was limited only to those sick or injured individuals who were usually cared for in homes through "private duty nursing." The nurse was customarily employed by the family, through a "registry," at the request of a physician. Often the physician would request a specific nurse for one of "his patients." In this relationship, there were four potentially competing ethical loyalties: patient, registry, physician, self.

Later, both patient care and nursing moved into hospitals. Nurses continued to be employed as private duty nurses, even within hospitals, until World War II, after which nurses predominantly became employees of the hospital rather than the patient or patient's family. Now the nurse faced loyalties to an institution instead of a registry, a physician whom the nurse may or may not have known, the patient, and self. In the days of registries and, subsequently, in hospitals, nurses could be blackballed, sometimes solely at the request of a physician, sometimes for reasons unrelated to practice. This heightened to need for nurses to be "loyal" to the physician. It has only been in recent years that a physician could not march into a nursing administration office and demand the firing of a particular nurse. Such power placed nurses in a terrible position—not only did the nurse have to "obey" and not oppose a physician, but the nurse also had to "please" the physician with a proper attitude of deference. Loyalty to the patient could be jeopardized where nurses believed their livelihood to be at stake. In addition, nurses were expected to serve, sometimes without remuneration, placing yet another strain on the nurse's loyalty to the patient. And yet, nursing, in its literature and its practice consistently articulated a primary commitment to the patient. After the 1950s, health care, or more specifically, illness care, has become far more complex than in the days of the inception of modern nursing in the United States in the 1870s. Nursing has moved out of diploma programs and into colleges and universities, and uniform mandatory registration and licensure has been instituted across the nation.

Both medicine and nursing have developed specialties and subspecialties, so the patients (and the nurses) now deal with a battalion of physicians in each case. Third party payors have entered into the mix, including both insurance companies and government agencies. Unionization and collective bargaining on behalf of nurses has increased. Accrediting bodies, both for institutions and for professions, have also become a part of the system. Many formerly independent hospitals have either gone out of business or coalesced into multihospitals and multiagency megacompanies. Restrictions may now be placed on care for economic rather than clinical reasons. And, importantly, there has been a rise in technological interventions available and both rising costs and access to care has become a problem for many. Increasingly, "competition" between ethical "loyalties" for nurses have become ever more robust and complex. In addition, though illness care remains the focus of the "healthcare system," there is an awareness of the importance of preventive care.

Preventive care was not greatly valued until an understanding of disease etiology came about in the 1870s and 1980s when Robert Koch and Louie Pasteur worked out the germ theory. Florence Nightingale, who was at Scutari and the Crimea in 1854, had no scientific knowledge of the germ theory, nor did she support the idea later, yet she was among the first to value prevention and to see the benefit of keeping people out of hospitals, which were often defined then as death houses. Before she became the famous "Lady with the Lamp," she had become convinced that improved public health measures were the royal road to making Britain a healthier nation, and became known in London social circles for her panoramic expertise in this field. Her much read *Notes on Nursing* (Nightingale, 1860) and her reorganization of the military health system reflected this knowledge and her value of disease prevention. Her vision enlarged the definition of the patient role and redefined the nursing role.

Once modern public health systems were established in the United Kingdom and the United States, the roles and functions of nurses expanded to include not only the sick, but the well; and not only individuals, but groups of people; with emphasis on cleanliness, vaccination, and prenatal and well-baby care. Though the nurse's role had expanded, the professional and ethical emphasis continued to be on the "patient," who might now be a family unit, a group, a community, or an individual.

In her book, *Nursing Ethics*, the American nurse Isabel Hampton Robb wrote:

I want to emphasize the fact that the nursing for all patients—rich or poor, in the hospital or in their own houses—is in the main identical... From the very outset let her [the nurse] determine that she will be no respecter of persons, but will treat all her patients with impartiality. While in the hospital, the nurse should always make it her rule to think of every patient—even the poorest and most unattractive—not as a mere case, interesting only from a scientific standpoint, but as an individual sick human being, whose wishes, fancies and peculiarities call for all the consideration possible at her hands. (Robb, 1900; pp. 213–14)

These words demonstrate the central place of all patients, with unique and individual attributes, in nursing and nursing ethics.

In each ANA Code since the first one in 1950, the patient, whether individual, family, group, or community, has been at the center of the nursing profession's ethics. That is still the case today, but life in general, nursing practice in particular, and the structure of the healthcare system, have become far more complex and the new ANA Code reflects these changes.

Thinking Behind This Provision

Though it has been the case that, throughout modern nursing in the United States, nurses have been morally obligated to put the patient first, the previous versions of the Code commingled this obligation with others. The Task Force for the Revision of the Code felt strongly that the primacy of the patient was of sufficient importance, historicity, and priority that it necessitated an emphatic and unequivocal statement in the provisions. Thus, the previous Provision 2 was bumped to third place and the duty to the patient placed second.

Historically, nurses had ethical obligations that placed emphasis on attending to the patients' needs, and yet the context of nursing was not necessarily supportive of this obligation. Today, the nurse's ethical obligation to the patient, first, is even more complex to negotiate. Our present day ethics has moved from a fairly recent physician-oriented, paternalistic model in which physicians, using the ethical principle of nonmaleficence or "do no harm," knew what was "best for the patient." As nursing expanded its educational offerings, developed specialized practice areas, escalated its research, and even developed forms of independent practice, nurses generally moved into the realm of independent nursing functions while retaining the so-called dependent functions of carrying out medical orders. In recognizing its own right to participate in decision making and formulate plans of patient care, nursing moved to ethics that recognized patient's rights, including the right to know and discuss their health status and make healthcare decisions. Simultaneously, nurses began coming to a greater awareness of "nursing rights," particularly as they related to the delivery of high-quality health care. This changed ethics model functions in the midst of increased clinical complexities that include economic constraints and managed care environments. This does not mean that nurses see patients (or themselves) as sidelined by events and priorities, but it does mean that nurses must learn to deal with economic pressures that may compete with moral values or with patients' rights. The patients and their rights must remain central. At the same time, ethical obligation to the patient is primary, but it is not the sole ethical obligation.

In this latest edition of the Code, Provision 5 has been added with the potential of creating additional ethical conflicts between the needs and rights of the patient and the nurse as it describes a nurse's duty to self. The function of duties to self is not some sort of entitlement; it is care for the self in such as way as to enable nurses to fulfill other moral duties. At times, nurses have, wrongly, placed their own needs before those of the patient in situations as simple as failing to confront a physician colleague who is indifferent or worse to the needs of the patient. Such situations, and others like it, that present the nurse with possible conflicting obligations raise several questions. First, does the nurse's primary obligation always mean a focus on the patient, as has historically been the case, even to the harm of the nurse? A "no" answer to this would require a strong ethical argument to support it. There may be an exception to this primary commitment, but a nurse would have to think long and hard about the ethical reason to act on this exception. Importantly, even in situations of conflicting moral claims, where the nurse must act in a morally self-regarding manner, the nurse must never abandon the patient. This means that if one nurse cannot, on ethical grounds, engage in some treatment, activity, or procedure, then another nurse or caregiver must be found who does not object to such involvement.

Nurses have multiple ethical obligations, sometimes competing, sometimes conflicting, including those to the patient, the organization or institution in which they work, other healthcare professionals, and the nursing profession. Today, as nursing becomes increasingly entrepreneurial, a nurse's own "business priorities" could conceivably come into conflict with the needs of the patient. Sometimes the nurse must decide to whom she or he owes a primary obligation (Davis et al, 1997). The Code says the primary obligation is to the patient. Nursing work always occurs in some social structure and this fact can make it difficult always to put the patient first in a nurse's ethical obligations. When nurses focus on what they think will be the consequences of an ethical act, sometimes they may need courage (a virtue) in order to act. They also need to draw support from the nursing community within which they work. In order to make this provision of the Code have full meaning, nursing leaders in all care giving settings will need to create environments in which candid, reflective, and open ethical discussions can take place.

How do nurses think about an ethical problem to arrive at some conclusion that they believe to be the ethically right action? Ethical decision making requires knowledge and refection including knowledge of clinical practice, institutional policies and procedures, the field of ethics, the Code of Ethics for Nurses, and an understanding of the self and one's own values. While the patient remains at the center of this thinking, other people need to be considered, including the same self-consideration on the part of the nurse.

Applying the Provision:
The Nurse-Patient Relationship

The nurse–patient relationship creates the basic unit in which much of nursing practice and ethics occurs. A nurse's ethical sensitivity is the first requirement in the application of this provision that places the patient at its center. Sometimes, nurses define a problem as a clinical one without seeing the ethical aspects in it. If the ethical issues that exist are missed, then that part of the situation is not attended to by the nurse. If the nurse is clinically competent, but ethically insensitive or oblivious, then this provision will not have a part in the decision making and actions that are needed to deal with the whole patient situation. If nurses are sensitive to the ethical issues or concerns involved in a given situation, the next step is them to pay attention to their own reactions to this situation. This reaction informs the nurse that something is wrong or missing ethically. This sensitivity and intuitive reaction comes from our values and socialization as children into adulthood. This informal, basic ethics education is further developed in nursing school where students are taught and socialized into the values and ethics of nursing. Sometimes, these values are deep enough that we may not be aware of them until they arise in a specific situation. It is at this point that one needs to examine both the situation and the reaction that one has had to it more closely.

To examine the ethics of the situation, one needs some way of viewing the ethical issues. This calls for knowledge of the clinical situation, the people involved, and the patient's values and wishes. Nurses can use ethical principles, such as respect for patient autonomy, nonmaleficence (the noninfliction of harm), beneficence (or doing good), justice, truth telling, and promise keeping (Beauchamp and Childress, 2001). To use these principles, one needs some understanding of what each of these principles mean and how they interact. This requires basic ethics education. For example, the ethical principle "respect for autonomy" is very important, but it is not absolute. This means that, in some limited and carefully thought-out situations, patient autonomy can be overridden in the service of another, more stringent, ethical principle, to do no harm. In using the ethical principle "do no harm" to override a patient's autonomous choice, health professionals need to be very clear that it is the patient who is being kept from harm and not the caregiving staff. Additionally, it is so much "easier" simply to tell people what they should do than to explain their clinical situation to them and have them participate in the decision making process. This is true whether the patient is an individual, family, group, or community.

But creating easy situations for healthcare professionals is not what ethics is about. Nurses use ethical principles such as "respect for autonomy," "do not harm," and "doing good" as they engage in ethical reflection and deliberation. They also use aspects of "caring ethics" that is developing as an alternative ethical theory. These aspects are: attentiveness, responsibility, competence, and responsiveness.

Ethical problems often relate to the tensions between responsibilities, as well as the multiple commitments of people who live or work in a network of relationships. It becomes necessary to interpret the different view points of all those involved with an ethical problem. It is also necessary to understand that our own values, obligations, loyalties, and ideals arise from multiple sources, as do those of others. In situations with people from cultures that differ from that of the nurse, value and obligation structures that come into play can be further complicated. Values underlie our ethical analyses, choices, and actions. Not all values are shared; thus, different people may choose or act in ways that would not be the choices or actions of the nurse What may seem strange to one person may be perfectly reasonable to another, given that person's world view, culture, and values (Davis, 2003).

When nurses deal with a group or community as the patient, notions of justice may come into play. Where resources are limited or managed, the principle of distributive justice is particularly important. Distributive justice refers to the sharing of burdens and benefits in the allocation of resources, sometimes, but not always, under conditions of scarcity or rationing. Customarily terms such as "fair," "equitable," "just," and "fitting" are used with regard to "justice" in the distribution of resources. The nurse needs to think through how to be fair in any issue of resource allocation, including the nurse's skill and attention or time.

In thinking through ethically problematic situations, the nurse will need to answer some questions. What, if any anything, should I do to be ethical in this situation? Why?

Thinking about these basic questions may help in this process:

- What do I know about this patient situation?

- What do I know about the patients' values and moral preferences?

- What assumptions am I making that need more data to clarify?

- What are my own feelings (and values) about the situation and how might they be influencing how I view and respond to this situation?

- Are my own values in conflict with those of the patient?

- What else do I need to know about this case and where can I obtain this information?

- What can I never know about this case?

- Given my primary obligation to the patient, what should I do to be ethical?

Case Example 1

The 87-year-old patient has end-stage lung cancer and is nearing the terminal phase, though not yet considered "terminally ill" for the purposes of admission to hospice. He tells the nurse that he is tired and does not want any more treatment, but he does want to be "kept comfortable." He indicates that he is tired of trying to fight the cancer and feels that his present life has no quality. Also, he says, "I have lived a good, long life and I am ready to go." His adult children have had a conference with the physician and said they want everything done for their father. The physician tends to go along with these adult children. What does the nurse need to know about this clinical situation? What are the values and obligations at stake in this case? What values or obligations should be affirmed and why? How might that be done? ∎

Case Example 2

The 32-year-old patient is in persistent vegetative state and has been for some years. The patient's outdated advance directive is confusing on the issue of food and fluid, though clear about not wanting to be on a ventilator if she were in a coma. Her husband wants the feeding tube removed, but is unable to say that it would have been the patient's wish. He says that it is his decision for her. Her two adult siblings and parents reject this as a possibility because, they say, "human life is sacred" and that their daughter believed this. They say their daughter is alive and should receive nursing care, including feeding. The healthcare team does not know what to do ethically and fear being sued by either the husband, siblings, or the parents. What do you need to know about this clinical situation? What are the values and obligations at stake in this case? What values or obligations should be affirmed and why? How might that be done? ■

Case Example 3

The national nursing shortage problem has arrived at the local hospital and the Vice President for Nursing is having difficulties staffing all units adequately, even though two units have been closed altogether. She can either spread the nurses around the hospital and keep all the remaining units open with fewer nurses on each unit than is really safe, or she can close some additional units and place those nurses on other units to have an adequate nursing staff. This choice would be safer for admitted patients, but other patients could not be admitted due to closed units. In order to reason through this problem of resource allocation, the nurse administrator must rely on the ethical principles of justice, nonmaleficence, and beneficence. This VP for Nursing must consider the welfare of the institution, the nursing staff, and the patients. How would you assess this situation morally. In your ethical analysis, what would be acceptable options? What would not be acceptable? How might the Code for Nurses inform the VP's decision? What choice of action might promote the most good while creating the least harm? ■

Case Example 4

This year there is a severe shortage of influenza vaccine. The policy from the Central Health Department is to restrict this vaccine only to pregnant women and people who are 60 years of age or older until such time as additional vaccine might become available. The potential availability of additional vaccine in the coming weeks is uncertain. The nurse himself is worried about exposure to the flu from the clinic population as he is at higher risk of exposure than the general population. Due to the nursing shortage, he is the only "shot nurse" for this extremely busy vaccination clinic. His is 35. He is considering giving himself the vaccine, or asking a colleague to do it. If you were that nurse, how would you reason, ethically, about taking the vaccine yourself? What arguments would you make for and against taking the vaccine? What do you believe to be the strongest argument? How might the Code assist you in making a decision? ■

Summary

The patient—individual, family, group, community—stands at the center of nursing's ethics. There are several ways for nurses to reason through ethical problems to reach an ethical solution. First, nurses need to be aware that each situation is an ethical problem and then they need to obtain as much information as possible about the clinical facts as well as ascertaining the values and wishes of the patient or the patient's surrogate in order to think the problem through. There is a body of knowledge, nursing ethics, that they can use for this decision making process. Two nursing ethics approaches were briefly mentioned above—principle based ethics and caring ethics (Davis et al, 2006).

The patient, broadly defined, will remain at the center of nursing ethics; however, nurses will continue to face ethical problems that they need to think through carefully using their Code of Ethics for Nurses and other sources of knowledge.

References

Beauchamp, T., and J. Childress. 2001. *Principles of Biomedical Ethics*. 5th ed. New York: Oxford University Press.

Davis, A.J. 2003. International Nursing Ethics: Context and Concerns. In *Approaches to Ethics*, V. Tschudin, ed., pp. 95–104. London: Butterworth-Heinemann.

Davis, A.J., M.A. Aroskar, J. Liaschenko, and T. Drought. 1997. *Ethical Dilemmas and Nursing Practice*. 4th ed. Stamford, CT: Appleton & Lange.

Davis, A.J., V. Tschudin, and L. deRaeve, eds. 2006. *Essentials of Teaching and Learning Nursing Ethics: Perspectives and Methods*. London: Elsevier.

Nightingale, F. 1860. *Notes on Nursing: What It Is and What It Is Not*. London: Harrison & Sons.

Robb, I.H. 1900. *Nursing Ethics: For Hospitals and Private Use*, pp. 213–214. Cleveland: E.C. Koeckert, Publisher.

Suggested Reading

Benjamin, M.J., and J. Curtis. 1991. *Ethics in Nursing*, 3rd ed. New York: Oxford University Press.

Tuckett, A.G. 2004. Truth-telling in clinical practice and the arguments for and against: A review of the literature. *Nursing Ethics* 11(5): 500–13.

Volbrecht R.M. 2002. *Nursing Ethics: Communities in Dialogue*. Old Tappan, NJ: Prentice Hall.

About the Author

Anne J. Davis, PhD, DS, MS, RN, FAAN, and Professor Emerita, taught at the University of California for 34 years. Beginning in 1962, Dr. Davis's career focused on international work with appointments in Israel, India, Nigeria, Ghana, Kenya, Japan, Korea, China, and Taiwan. These rich experiences led to the development of her over-riding interest in cultural diversity and nursing ethics. She is a graduate of Emory University in Atlanta (BS, Nursing), Boston University (MS, Psychiatry), and University of California, Berkeley (PhD, Higher Education). Dr. Davis has been the recipient of numerous awards, including an honorary Doctor of Science from Emory University and election as a Fellow in the American Academy of Nursing.

Provision Three

The nurse promotes, advocates for, and strives to protect the health, safety, and rights of the patient.

Provision Three

John G. Twomey, PhD, PNP

As a modern document, the 2001 Code of Ethics tends to be less directive than other professional codes. A review of the codes of ethics of other allied health professionals (for example, physical therapists and speech and language specialists) reveals that these professions tend be much more prescriptive in language about what is allowable or discouraged behaviors in their respective health professions. This can cause some questioning from nurses who believe that a code of ethics should be rather directive. The Code of Ethics Task Force deliberately created a code that focused on moral concepts that undergird the profession and did not attempt to make statements that would bind the individual nurse in all situations to a single course of action.

Even a deliberative document that states as its goal the provision of a moral framework must provide some specific behaviors for the members to consistently adhere to. In Provision 3, the reader will find language and some guidelines for the nurse who is working in any practice arena.

The Task Force recognized that, even in a document that was fairly revolutionary in its writing, it was necessary to bring forward concepts and language that the members of the profession would recognize from the last and previous Codes. More importantly, the authors had to honor many of the traditional moral beliefs and behaviors that nurses had been taught and were familiar with. So in this provision, concrete terms are used with updated nuances in the interpretive statements. Concepts such as protection of privacy and concern for subjects in healthcare research, as well as the professional values nurses have developed regarding dealing with impaired colleagues are taken from their separate places in the 1985 Code and grouped together here in Provision 3.[1]

To begin with, what are unifying concepts that help fit Provision 3 and its interpretive statements properly into the Code? First of all, the title of the Provision contains language that focuses the nurse's actions on encounters with patients. This Provision finalizes the process begun in Provisions 1 and 2, declaring to all that the ultimate moral duties of professional nurses involve working with people who need nursing care. The first three Provisions reiterate what nursing, through the American Nurses Association, has been stating for decades: When individuals need nursing care, only a professional registered nurse is educationally and morally capable of providing such care. This is a claim that can be traced directly back to Florence Nightingale and her successors, such Adelaide Nutting, Lavinia Dock, and others. Thus, our updated Code serves to link nurses practicing in the 21st century to our roots two centuries ago.[2]

But historical traditions need some substance that is recognized by the profession and its members if the legacy given to us is going to be meaningful in today's practice. The conceptual model that Provision 3 follows is one that nursing has embraced for many years. The phrase used in this provision *"to protect"* is deliberately chosen because of its recognized place in nursing practice. As the nursing profession matured in the second half of the 20th century, its members embraced the concept of protection as a core part of nursing. The Task Force wanted to be very particular in its use of terms around protection. Once assumed to be defined within the concept of advocacy, the concept of protection is expanded in Provision 3 to include all patients. This concept is extended to not just those with diminished health capacities, but to all who encounter the nurse and need assistance to protect their universal health needs, including but not limited to protection of information, need for education about health, and protection from those healthcare providers who are incompetent and/or impaired. So protection takes on a comprehensive definition within the Code.

Before moving on to a discussion of each interpretive statement, there must also be some mention of the ethical basis for the ideas in the provision, as well as the overall values reflected within the concept of protection. The 2001 Code uses a variety of ethical theories and concepts to reflect the diverse moral beliefs that American nurses bring to their practice. Despite this diversity, there are some unifying themes that will be described within this reader. Provision 3 reflects the bioethical theory based on the use of *principles*.[3] This approach is probably the most widely used approach to bioethics among clinicians in the Western world and its specific primary principles are widely embraced in clinical practice and often by institutional bioethics committees as well. While the concept of protection fits well within the principle-based system, the reader must be clear about how a specific principle supports protection as it is described in the 2001 Code.

While many nurses would recognize the principle of *nonmaleficence*, which is often articulated as the duty of "the noninfliction of harm," it would be incorrect to attribute this principle as the theoretical root of Provision 3. Instead, the ethical principle of *respect for autonomy* drives this provision. Provisions 1 and 2 define a basic part of the nurse-patient relationship as respect for individuals, their dignity and worth. The moral foundation for this respect is grounded in the basic value of human dignity and in this sense the individual characteristics of the patient are irrelevant. All persons have worth and dignity. Indeed, what the nursing profession wants its members to do as part of this respect for autonomy is to preserve and safeguard it. An essential piece of autonomy is that those who possess it do so because they have, have had, or will develop the capacity to make decisions for and about themselves. Respect for autonomy is necessary because the nature of health and threats to it mean that the capacity to remain autonomous does not always remain fully intact. So Provision 3 uses a principled approach, through its protection of and respect for autonomy, as its ethical basis.

Privacy and Confidentiality: Interpretive Statements 3.1 and 3.2

The first two parts of this provision refer to safeguarding information. In the prior two versions of the Code, the concept of protecting the patient's personal information had been given an entire provision. Because the Task Force wanted to emphasize the concept of protection, it expanded the provision containing this concept to include situations where the need for safeguarding the patient may occur. This expansion resulted in Provision 3 being the longest in the 2001 Code.

To emphasize the complexity of protecting patient information, the definitions of privacy and confidentiality are separated and explained. Privacy relates to those aspects of a patient's life and information that he or she can control. It is that control that the nurse is charged with helping to preserve. Honoring a patient's privacy can be as simple as only asking questions that are clinically relevant, but can also extend to constructing policies that maintain privacy, such as hospital environment policies. Confidentiality is a term that refers to making sure that once a patient has shared personal information, such data is used only in ways that are authorized by the patient.

To provide an example of respect for privacy, consider the questions that arise if Mrs. Cummings comes to the surgical clinic for a preoperative breast surgery visit. During the visit and exam, the nurse notes a large bruise along her lower rib cage and she shares with the nurse that her husband inflicted it last night in a fight about the surgery. She explains that he does not want her to have prophylactic breast surgery after she tested positive for the BRCA1 gene mutation, which means she is at higher risk for breast cancer than the general population. After the nurse determines that the bruise has no physiological implications for surgery and that Mrs. Cummings has arranged to go to her sister's home for immediate post-op care, the nurse should agree when Mrs. Cummings' requests that no mention of the fight be placed in her medical record. That is her right and if she wishes to keep the information private, she may. Withholding this information from the medical record does not require that the nurse simply ignore what has happened. The nurse is obligated to review the nursing and health literature on domestic violence and to follow up in so far as the patient will permit. Additional assessment is called for. For instance, the nurse should ascertain whether this is a single episode or a habitual situation, whether children are at risk in the home, and so forth. This should not simply be dropped: The nurse may offer Mrs. Cummings additional options, such as referral to counseling, and may engage in patient education regarding domestic violence should such education not be resisted. In some states laws covering domestic violence mandate healthcare professionals to report even a suspicion of domestic violence that is discovered in the process of caregiving. These laws differ from state to state, but nurses need to be aware of these laws.

Contrast this example with the issue of confidentiality that the genetics nurse confronted when Mrs. Cummings originally requested the BRCA1 genetic test and stated that she did not want the result to be placed in her medical record, because she feared that she might face future discrimination in work or in obtaining life or health insurance if the test were positive. While this might appear again to be a request for privacy, it becomes an issue of confidentiality if the policy at the Breast Cancer Genetics Clinic is that all test results must be in a patient record, even if the patient pays for them personally. Now the nurse must discuss with Mrs. Cummings how the information will be preserved and limits to its protection, if she chooses to be tested at this particular clinic. While the duty to protect, here, is still owed to the patient, this example shows that the nurse must be very proactive in being aware of how information will be preserved and protected and in what ways.[4] Such a duty extends beyond the clinical encounter to efforts such as participating in establishing institutional policies or even state laws that that protect confidentiality. Thus, in this situation, the patient is protected by being informed in advance, and the nurse protects future patients by participating in policy formulation with regard to confidentiality of clinical information.

The interpretive statements on privacy and confidentiality are necessarily broad so that they can serve as useful guidance in a range of contexts and situations. The Code does not specify concrete and absolute rules about how to protect patient information in a "one rule fits all situations" approach. The complexity of this issue has recently been highlighted by the institution of the Health Information Portability Accountability Act and its Privacy Rule.[5] Nurses, like all healthcare providers, have had to attend in-service educational offerings about the implications of the Rule so that they can advise patients about who may access their health information. In the midst of the well-publicized efforts to implement the Rule, it must not be forgotten that medical information passes through many hands and the nurse is only one participant in the process of storing this data. Often the nurse's most significant contribution is to be able to advise the patient as to where their data will be stored, who will have access to it, and with whom it will be shared. This facilitates better decision making by the patient. In the prior example of Mrs. Cummings and her concern about her genetic test results, the nurse may be able to advise her that the clinic policy is that no information is released to employers or insurance companies unless she signs a release form. This policy would allow those in the health team to have access to necessary patient information while providing a certain level of protection that the patient can control.

Many policies exist to help patients to protect their health information. These policies may affect the ability of the nurse to carry out his or her ethical duties. Another factor that complicates this duty is that the duty to maintain confidentiality is not absolute. Specifically, in some instances when a third party may suffer harm if information discovered in the process of nursing care is withheld from the other involved individual, there may be a legal as well as a moral duty to protect the other person. It is incumbent upon the nurse to clarify the duty to protect and to understand both its moral and legal dimensions.

There is a related category of exceptions to absolute confidentiality. All states have mandatory reporting laws that the nurse must honor if child abuse or neglect is suspected and many jurisdictions have extended such limits to confidentiality to cases where nurses become privy to threats to the health and safety of elders.[6] What if the nurse is concerned about the safety of the patient's health after a clinical encounter? Can the information that the diabetic patient does not want the nurse to report to the clinic physician that she has stopped testing her blood sugar be withheld? In general, nurses cannot withhold information that would negatively impact patient safety or directly affect the quality of care. Information clearly related to the patient's care must be shared with the physician, but it is best if this information comes from the patient. In exploring the reasons why the patient has stopped testing her blood sugar, and why she does not wish this specific information disclosed to the physician, the nurse must assess the patient, ascertaining why she has stopped testing her blood sugar levels. Perhaps she has stopped for a simple and correctable reason (such as the cost of supplies). The nurse should then discuss with the patient the physician's need for this information and the serious consequences of withholding it. The patient should be urged and enabled by the nurse to share this key information.

Where clinical care is compromised, the nurse has a duty to advise the patient not to withhold this information, and to explain that the nurse has a duty to maintain the quality of patient care, including disclosing the information as a last resort. In addition to counseling the patient that disclosing the information would be essential to her safe clinical management, the nurse could consult the immediate supervisor or perhaps ultimately the institution's bioethics committee if assistance is needed in resolving conflicts of this nature.

Other examples of limits on confidentiality include public health laws that mandate reporting of certain health conditions such as an infectious disease, like tuberculosis, within a community. On the other hand, there are some special cases. where specific medical information, such as HIV status, cannot be shared without specific state policies to the contrary,[7] no matter how high you judge the potential threat to a third party.

Protection of Participants in Research: Interpretive Statement 3.3

The 1976 Code for Nurses included guidelines for the nurse working with participants in research in its seventh provision, which addressed the role of the nurse in promoting the scientific knowledge of the profession. The relocation of this concern to the third provision in the current Code reflects the increased activity of nurses as nurse-researchers, or as members of a research team, and the increase in research activity in all settings, including community hospitals and agencies, not just "research institutions." Patients are more likely today than ever before to be faced with a decision whether or not to take part in research that might be related to their condition or care. Because of the complexity of options that occur when research is combined with care, inclusion of this interpretive statement under this provision focuses the primary role of the nurse in all research activity on insuring that subjects are aware of the potential risks and are protected to the greatest extent possible from those risks. Nurse researchers are also obligated to reduce risk in their studies to the lowest level possible.

This interpretive statement has two paragraphs. The first focuses on duties that any nurse who is in a relationship with a research participant must carry out. Focusing on the concept of informed consent as a significant tool in facilitating the ability of the research subject to make decisions, the nurse is identified as a key participant in the ongoing consent process. Note that consent is, in fact, ongoing and not a one-time activity. In effect, the nurse who has an ongoing relationship with the patient-as-research-subject is given the heavy responsibility of assessing the person's ability to understand the ongoing dynamic of the research process. This contrasts with the research team, which often spends little time with the participant and often do not make ongoing evaluations of the level of the subject's understanding.[8]

Consider the following scenario that many nurses encounter. An elderly man is admitted to your unit after a hip replacement procedure. During his stay, you note that every day at noon, a nurse comes to the unit and administers an oral medication. You inquire about the medicine and the nurse explains that the man is on a double-blind, placebo-controlled research trial to study the effect of norepinephrine on depression in people from 65 to 90 years. You read the protocol and note that it employs a crossover methodology and because your patient is ending his sixth week on the study medication, in two days, he will be switched to the other blinded medication arm. That afternoon, as you do some post-operative care with the man, you mention the research study. He smiles and his wife notes, "We're so happy they asked him to be in the study. He's improved so much. We're so lucky that he got the right medication." You ask how they feel about the upcoming switch to the other medication and they look at you with surprise. The wife says, "No, no. The study was to find out what was the best for him and now we know."

This patient and his wife are showing signs of a phenomenon known as *therapeutic misconception*. This occurs when a research subject fails to understand that the goal of a research protocol is not to provide him with individual benefit and assumes that the job of the researcher is the same as the caregiver—to give him only those interventions that will improve his health.[9] In this situation, the family clearly anticipates that the patient will be kept on the medication that helped him and do not understand the change of medication that may not provide the same effects and actually may result in a reversal of his improvement. Nurses have a role in protecting patients whether involved in research or in clinical trials, and to advocate that all provisions for informed consent be observed. The research nurse or the nurse member of a research team is in relationship with the patient-as-human-subject and the family and is expected to assure that the participant's active and consistent interpretation of the goals of the research or clinical trial is clear.

If this were your patient, this part of Provision 3 imparts an imperative to act that provides several options. One is to discuss the protocol with the family, but that is probably only a beginning. Because the patient obviously signed the consent form without a full understanding of the protocol, the researchers must be notified and asked to meet with the patient and his wife to review the details of the study. If the nurse is unsatisfied that the explanation given to the patient is complete and understandable, she should express her concerns to the principal investigator of the study. If the nurse's concerns are not resolved, the nurse should then contact the facility's human subject's protection committee or Institutional Review Board (IRB) that originally approved the details of the research, including the wording of the consent form, and express her misgivings.

The second paragraph contains more information about the research review and protection process. Since 1976, nurses have become much more involved in the conduct of nursing research, as the number of nursing doctoral programs has increased and the National Institute of Nursing Research has opened at the National Institutes of Health. From a regulatory perspective, the *Belmont Report* of The National Commission for the Protection of Human Subjects of Biomedical and Behavioral Research provided the theoretical basis for the regulations published in 1983 that govern human subjects research in the United States.[10] While most codes of ethics for health professions mention the ethical conduct of research, the more extended detail of this provision makes the Code of Ethics for Nurses unique in the attention given to this topic.

The interpretive statement can be misinterpreted, however. By continuing to identify the object of research as a patient, it may appear to have less relevance for healthy subjects whom the nurse may encounter. But even the short relationships formed in the outpatient setting should not inhibit the nurse from advising subjects about their rights as human subjects. With regard to children, parents do not give *consent* (despite the label on the form) since *consent* refers only to one's own agreement. Parents almost always must provide permission for their children to be research subjects, and the *Code of Federal Regulations (FCR)* requires that researchers "solicit the assent of children" who are capable of assenting. Morally, a child's refusal of assent should be considered binding. The FCR further states that "if the IRB determines that the… intervention or procedure involved in the research holds out a prospect of direct benefit that is important to the health or well-being of the children *and is available only in the context of research*, the assent of the children is not a necessary condition for proceeding with the research" [italics added]. In addition, the FCR states that "if the IRB determines that a research protocol is designed for conditions or for a subject population for which parental or guardian permission is *not a reasonable requirement to protect the subjects (for example, neglected or abused children)*, it may waive the consent requirements… provided an appropriate mechanism for protecting the children who will participate as subjects in the research is substituted… " [italics added]. From the perspective of ethics, in any research setting, even young children should be included in the research enrollment process by educating them about their participation to the level of their developmental understanding and capacity.[11]

Standards and Review Mechanisms: Interpretive Statement 3.4

This important interpretive statement could be placed under several of the provisions in the Code. Here the development and maintenance of basic competencies for nursing is discussed. In addition, there follows the description of basic competencies with an accounting of activities that more experienced nurses should be engaged in. Nurses in varied roles must participate in or facilitate the involvement of others in activities that contribute to superior patient care. While the activities listed under this interpretive statement certainly could be used to support other provisions, such as those later in the Code that focus more on the professional status of nursing itself, the Task Force decided to reinforce that these activities are not just self-protecting or self-promoting, but are patient-centered actions that rightfully belong under the provision that focuses on protection of patient rights and well-being.

The first paragraph in this interpretive statement has a seemingly straightforward directive: All nurses, whether educators, administrators, or clinicians share equal responsibilities to ensure that the daily care provided to patients comes from nurses who have had to meet standards that the professional nursing group has agreed upon. Educators must make certain that their curricula contain the theoretical and clinical knowledge necessary for novices to enter the profession as competent beginning practitioners. Nursing administrators must also assess and provide for the ongoing educational needs of clinicians to move into the increasingly complex world of today's healthcare institutions.

The background message in this paragraph is that no matter what their specific activity and responsibility, nurses practice nursing care and that all nursing care is patient-centered. The American Nurses Association, which sponsors the Code of Ethics, and its federal and state units, has a central theme that it represents all registered nurses. At a time when the needs of patients and healthcare organizations has spawned the need for increasing subspecialization within the profession, there has been a growth of specialty groups that claim to speak for their members, even to the point of writing their own standards and codes of ethics.[12] One result of this trend has been for the "bedside" nurses, providing "generalist" care, to believe that they are not well represented by an organization that is run by highly educated nurses who seem distant from any patient care. The Task Force wanted to reiterate that the Code is for all registered nurses, in all specialties, in all roles, whether their work affects patients directly or indirectly. So the nurse educator who lectures on health policy is practicing nursing as well as the nurse supervisor who spends much time maintaining proper staffing levels. All nurses participate in weaving a tapestry of care that protects patients throughout their encounter with the healthcare system when in relationship with a nurse.

This philosophy of professional equality is carried forth in the second paragraph of the interpretive statement. While, again, designated nursing leaders have responsibility for maintaining access of their staff to the ongoing mechanisms of care promotion and review, it is both a right and responsibility of today's highly prepared nurse to participate in all institutional activities that affect patient care. Indeed, patient care is being carried out in the conference room when nurses, physicians, and other care providers meet to discuss and plan for new models of care delivery as well as completing reviews of current models. Nurses are expected to identify barriers to optimal patient care, nursing and otherwise, and step up and demand that such obstructions be eliminated, and work toward that end. Part of the ethical responsibility of today's highly educated registered nurses is to be active leaders in health care, not passive followers.

The final paragraph of this interpretive statement seems to have anticipated the recent Institute of Medicine report on patient morbidities related to healthcare system errors.[13] This section anticipates that conscientious nurses will at times recognize that patients have been exposed to harms because of suboptimal practices within the healthcare institution and that the nurse must be an agent of change to protect other patients suffering from similar, preventable errors. Nurses have an ethical obligation to identify the source of the error and take steps to eliminate it, specifically through established institutional pathways. A specific proscription of this interpretive statement is on keeping the knowledge of the error or questionable practice secret. The following vignette shows the difficult issues that this part of the statement identifies.

Case Example 1

You have been hired as a newly graduated inpatient nurse practitioner. You feel that your graduate program and its preceptors had provided you with a modern, progressive set of practice skills. As you get oriented, you are told that people here work on a team and may often be providing care to patients who are shared with other providers. That is not a problem most of the time, but you note that patients who have been worked up and have their care plan written primarily by nurse Virginia are not being cared for by state-of-the-art protocols and sometimes are being handled in ways that are invalidated by the nursing research literature. You are not sure what to do, for Virginia is one of the senior nurses and, though a peer, is crotchety and doesn't communicate well in team meetings. ■

In this vignette, there is reason to believe that patients are at risk of injury either directly or by failure to adhere to current standards of practice. Harm has not yet occurred, but you anticipate that it may. Does the new nurse practitioner have a duty to intervene? If so, how should the nurse practitioner's efforts be directed?

The new nurse practitioner clearly has an ethical obligation to the patients on this unit, even if they are not her direct responsibility. She has graduated with a working knowledge of state-of-the-art clinical practice and has recognized that such practices are being withheld from the patients on her unit. The issue is what steps should she take? Initially, concerns should be expressed to the nurse directly and she should be given the opportunity to discuss this and to change if needed. The Code is not a document to detail the specific steps to be taken, but the interpretive statement makes plain that processes should be in place from an administrative standpoint for the nurse to go to a supervisor, if she believes that Virginia proves unreceptive to suggestions about possible changes to her practice. If the direct supervisor does not facilitate any intervention, then nurses in higher levels of leadership should be approached. Intermediate steps could be to hold in-service programs on current practices for the entire staff, establish institutional standards of practice, and peer review, and hope that Virginia responds with some changes.

This paragraph of interpretive statement section 3.4 introduces one of the most important topics contained within the Code. The issue of self-oversight by the nursing profession is very complex, being interwoven among all of the many agencies responsible for evaluation of nursing practice. The intricacies involved in oversight of nurses are part of the ethical behaviors of a profession and its members. Interpretive statement section 3.4 begins to detail the ways that nurses may be involved in such oversight, noting that most errors are a result of both human behavior and environmental factors and that any remediation efforts must address both of these aspects. But is also makes it clear, as do the last two sections of this interpretive statement, that individual nurses are responsible for seeing that such remediation does take place.

Acting on Questionable Practices and Addressing Impaired Practice: Interpretive Statements 3.5 and 3.6

Provision 3 is the longest of the nine provisions in the Code, and fully half of the provision is taken up with ethical guidelines for protecting the patient through taking steps to remediate poor practice. There are several probable reasons for such a commitment to patient advocacy on the part of nurses and such a dedicated statement to the public about these issues. These reasons include the constant skilled presence of the nurse in the patient's care, the close and intimate nature of the nurse–patient relationship, the ability of the nurse to observe and assess the patient's strengths and vulnerabilities, and the complexity of the healthcare system that make it difficult for patients to navigate the system or even to advocate for themselves. Another reason is that, traditionally, the provision of nursing has been ill-controlled by the profession, so that nursing care is delivered by many people, some with minimal qualifications, but the public has been unable to discern such differences in who actually is or is not a registered nurse. Another reason is that despite licensure laws, the provision of nursing has often been controlled by employers, who can allow anyone to wear scrubs, carry a stethoscope, and provide care associated with a nurse without any identification beyond wearing a tag with a first name on it. This can and does confuse the image and expectations of the public about nursing care.

Finally, the nursing profession has been unable to elevate, or even make consistent, the educational requirements for nurses. The effect is that nursing represents the largest group of healthcare professionals, but the group is a loosely organized collection of people with multiple backgrounds and skills. It is not surprising that the profession has great difficulty implementing consistent standards of care when such care cannot be assumed to be within the capabilities of the less well-educated and prepared caregivers who provide nursing care.

Provision 4 addresses the ethical aspect of the delegation of nursing care. This provision, specifically these two sections, make firm, unmistakable statements that say that nurses will protect their patients from direct, unprofessional care. This is the professional organization adamantly taking responsibility, through its individual members, for stopping in its tracks any behaviors that threaten patient safety

Interpretive Statements 3.5 and 3.6 contain much similar language. Comparable content involves identification of possibly dangerous behavior by an individual nurse, the realization that the behavior must be addressed, and pathways to do so. There is a hierarchy of actions that a nurse can take that begins internally through consultation with supervisors and moves up the administrative chain. If no resolution results from following internal processes and the behavior continues, then the nurse is encouraged to go outside the institution to other agencies that govern both patient care and professional nursing. The specific agencies to be consulted depend upon the nature of the state structure for oversight of health care and professional behavior. They would generally include the bureau of professional licensure, boards of quality assurance, or a board of health. Your state nursing association can also provide guidance and one should not hesitate to approach them, even if one is not a member. Finally, in some instances, reporting is mandated to state agencies, sometimes by the nurse directly and sometimes through a particular institutional unit. Here, the nurse needs to be familiar with state and county regulations and institutional procedures and policies. Review the following case and contrast it to Case Example 1.

Case Example 2

You are making a home visit to a patient who was discharged after having a stroke and falling. This fall caused a hip fracture and the patent still has significant pain, but you believe that he should be able to begin more ambulation in his home. You review his level of narcotic pain medication that has been charted as given several times a day by one of the visiting nurses. As you begin your assessment, the patient complains of excessive pain and wishes to stop the ambulation exercises you are doing with him. You determine that he is having significant pain and ask him if he thinks that he needs more medicine. He says," I haven't taken any medicine since last week except Tylenol. That's all the nurse says I need." By your assessment, the patient is clear, aware, and not forgetful. You then examine all his medications and find that even though prescribed, there are no narcotics, only Tylenol. ∎

What are your responsibilities to this patient and your profession? There are significant differences in the last two cases. The first case involves subtle but real differences in care performance, but such differences might only be apparent to members of the nursing profession. Also, unless Virginia's behavior hurts a patient and results in a malpractice case, it will not draw the interest of outside authorities. The actions described in Case Example 2 are much different. Not only has the patient been injured, there is strong circumstantial evidence that a serious crime may have been committed in the theft of narcotics. There are also reasonable indications that other patients may also be at risk from this unnamed nurse because it is possible, but not certain, that the nurse who may be stealing the narcotics, may also be using these narcotics and may be practicing while impaired.

There is no leeway available to the nurse in this situation. Interpretive Statements 3.5 and 3.6 are clear that in the first case, a nurse can approach Virginia privately to attempt to change her behavior. However, in the latter case, the potentially criminal nature of the actions of the nurse takes such discretion away. An immediate report must be made to the supervisors and the situation pursued officially. In the case of the theft of narcotics, a report must be made to civil authorities and possibly to the nursing or other boards (depending upon state laws) through the appropriate institutional or agency procedures for reporting outside the agency. In addition, a police report may be in order. A tougher case, from an ethical perspective, may be presented in a scenario such as in the following case.

Case Example 3

You work closely with several people at your small clinic and have started meeting socially to have a few drinks. You notice one of your fellow nurses, Brad, tends to drink more than the rest of the group. He lives nearby, walks home, and never seems abusive, so you never mention it until one day you return from lunch and you see Brad leaving a bar. In the clinic, you return a patient record to Brad and you smell liquor on his breath. He takes the record, smiles, and says, "Thanks. I needed this record. I'm seeing her in ten minutes." What concerns do you have as you return to your desk? The quality of Brad's patient care has never been questioned and patients always compliment him. What professional obligations do you have and how should they be carried out? ■

Interpretive Statement 3.6 infers that if you clearly believe that if Brad is impaired, then you have an obligation to report his condition to a superior. Of course, while the primary goal in both Case Examples 2 and 3 is patient protection, a secondary goal is to provide the involved nurses with necessary services to help overcome any impairment affecting performance. The difference is in how imminent any actions must be. The former case obviously needs immediate action. But how quickly, or cautiously, must the nurse act in Brad's case? Interpretive statement 3.6 does not provide a timeline, but notes that the profession, in addition to many healthcare and state professional organizations, is dedicated to providing remedial services to impaired professionals, not punishing them.

Any nurse who reads Interpretive Statements 3.5 and 3.6 will probably pause when it becomes apparent that the actions mandated within these sections could be very difficult to carry out. Part of most individual's professional identity is a sense of loyalty to one's fellow workers. Indeed, the moral principle of fidelity is a very important moral concept. But when fellow professionals act in ways that endanger patients as well as themselves or others, then obligations to the patient, the nursing profession, and the employing institution, supersede loyalty to a peer.

The Task Force recognized that the psychological pressure to protect a co-worker is not the only force that sometimes weakens the willingness of a nurse to confront behaviors that present immediate risk of harm to patients. Another powerful coercive factor is the fear of retaliation for "blowing the whistle" on those acting dangerously. It is not uncommon for a nurse to fear retaliation if she were to report that the actions of an established senior worker or even a superior who is incapacitated while at work or who practices unsafely.[14] Interpretive statement 3.6 places responsibility for those nurses in leadership positions within institutions and state licensure agencies to ensure that policies are in place to protect nurses who take the courageous step of reporting illegal, incompetent, or impaired practice.

In summary, Provision 3 of the Code of Ethics for Nurses continues the legacy of nurses having a moral basis for the traditional role of protecting patients' rights and interests, including the patients' physical safety. This provision grounds these ethical duties within the principle of respecting patient autonomy in conjunction with the nurse having a personal moral agency that guides nursing actions in ways that transcend institutional rules. This moral agency is embedded in the historical roles of nursing and is patient centered. The profession of nursing draws its moral force from the ethical actions of its individual members.

Endnotes

All online sources cited were accessed in December 2007.

1. Daly, B.J. 1999. Ethics: Why a new code? Code for Nurses. *American Journal of Nursing* 99(6): 64, 66.

2. Hamilton, D. 1994. Constructing the mind of nursing. *Nursing History Review* II: 3–28.

3. Beauchamp, T.L., and J.F. Childress. 2001. *Principles of Biomedical Ethics*, 5th ed. NY: Oxford University Press.

4. ISONG (International Society for Nurses in Genetics). 2007. Privacy and confidentiality of genetic information: The role of the nurse. http://www.isong.org/about/ps_privacy.cfm.

5. Artnak, K.E., and M. Benson. 2005. Evaluating HIPAA compliance: A guide for researchers, privacy boards, and IRBs. *Nursing Outlook* 53(2; Mar–Apr): 79–87 (31 ref).

6. Wieland, D. 2000. Abuse of older persons: An overview. *Holistic Nursing Practice* 14 (4; July): 40–50 (43 ref).

7. Herek, G.M., J.P. Capitanio, and K.F. Widaman. 2003. Stigma, social risk, and health policy: Public attitudes toward HIV surveillance policies and the social construction of illness. *Health Psychology,* 22(5; Sept): 533–40 (38 ref).

8. Veatch, R. 1987. *The Patient As Partner: A Theory of Human-Experimentation*

       Guide to the Code of Ethics for Nurses

Ethics. Bloomington, IN: Indiana University Press.

9. Appelbaum, P.S., C.W. Lidz, T. Grisso. 2004. Therapeutic misconception in clinical research: Frequency and risk factors. *IRB: A Review of Human Subjects Research* 26(2; Mar–Apr): 1–8.

10. Cassell, E.J. 2000. The principles of the Belmont Report revisited: How have respect for persons, beneficence, and justice been applied to clinical medicine? *Hastings Center Report* 30(4; Jul–Aug): 12–21 (3 ref).

11. Code of Federal Regulations, Title 45: Public Welfare, Part 46: Protection of Human Subjects, Rev. 23 June, 2005, Subpart D, Sections 46.401–409.

12. Broome, M.E., E. Kodish, G. Geller, L.A. Siminoff. 2003. Children in research: New perspectives and practices for informed consent. *IRB: Ethics and Human Research* 25(5; Sept–Oct): Sup. S20–25.

13. Anonymous. 2004. Keeping patients safe: Institute of Medicine looks at transforming nurses' work environment. *Quality Letter for Healthcare Leaders* 6(1): 9–11.

14. Ahern, K., S. McDonald. 2002. The beliefs of nurses who were involved in a whistleblowing event. *Journal of Advanced Nursing* 38(3; May): 303–309.

About the Author

John G. Twomey, PhD, PNP, is an Associate Professor at the Graduate Program in Nursing at the MGH Institute of Health Professions in Boston, Massachusetts. Dr. Twomey's doctoral work was in bioethics. He teaches bioethics and research and serves on several human subjects research protection committees. He has completed two National Institute of Nursing Research-supported postdoctoral fellowships in genetics. A member of the International Society of Nurses in Genetics, he does research in the area of the ethics of genetic testing of children. He is the editor of the Ethics Column in the Society's quarterly newsletter.

Provision
Four

The nurse is responsible and accountable for individual nursing practice and determines the appropriate delegation of tasks consistent with the nurse's obligation to provide optimum patient care.

Provision Four

Laurie A. Badzek, JD, LLM, MS, RN, NAP

Provision History

The framework for the inclusion of accountability and responsibility in the nursing ethical code is based upon many of the observations made by Florence Nightingale in the late 1800s. Nightingale dedicated her life to the advancement of the patient's physical, emotional, and environmental well-being. Nightingale's advances were the direct result of actions that improved quality care and the provision of education to those caring for persons of ill health. As detailed in *Notes on Nursing*, Nightingale recognized the importance of the choices made by a nurse in the daily care of patients and the accountability of the nurse for the outcomes of such care provided based on those choices.

The observations and documentations that Florence Nightingale made over a century ago recognized accountability as an essential characteristic of the nurse, and has enabled nursing to evolve into a strong, trusted profession, even in the face of current realities that complicate accountability and responsibility. Both the foresight and ingenuity Nightingale demonstrated resulted in an acknowledgement of the importance of accountability in providing high-quality care. The ethical accountability that nurses have today for the decisions and judgments they make can be directly traced to the writings of Nightingale.

In addition to a historical context dating back to Nightingale's time, accountability and responsibility for nursing care have a more recent context in the current laws related to licensure, contracts, and malpractice. Increasingly frequent lawsuits against healthcare providers that result in high monetary awards to injured plaintiffs make the application of nursing skill and judgment, including delegation of tasks, even more challenging. Nurses who lack competency or who fail to provide appropriate professional nursing care may be subject to legal liability as determined by the courts as well as licensure actions determined by the State Board of Nursing, which may potentially impact the ability of the nurse to practice. Nursing practices that reflect incompetence or other such failures of care does not meet the moral standards of the profession as embodied, in part, by this Code of Ethics.

Content of Provision 4

Provision 4 of the Code of Ethics for Nurses addresses the individual responsibilities and obligations of the nurse. Although much of nursing is collective and involves relationships with others, the inclusion of responsibility and accountability in the Code of Ethics for Nurses informs the nurse that responsibility for the individual actions and judgments made minute by minute, hour by hour, and daily over a lifetime of practice belongs solely to the individual nurse making the decisions. The Code of Ethics for Nurses helps define the relevant ethical obligations and duties nurses have not only to the public, but to themselves as well. Expanded knowledge of responsibility and accountability in nursing helps not only the profession, but also the general public to better understand the level to which nurses as professionals hold themselves and one another accountable and responsible for nursing practice.

Accountability is often identified as an attribute of a profession. The acceptance of accountability by the members of the profession is an implied contract with the public (Burkhart and Nathaniel, 2002). The Code of Ethics for Nurses sets forth explicitly the values and obligations of the nurse. The Code of Ethics for Nurses also provides a clear statement of what the public can expect from the nurse and the nursing community in relation to their professional practice.

Public confidence is a necessity for any profession and is especially important in health care where the services provided are of a personal and sensitive nature. Accountability of nurses for patient care outcomes enables them to hold an autonomous position in the healthcare industry. Nursing has time and again been selected as the most trusted profession in several national polls, including the Gallup Poll (2006), thus demonstrating that nursing as a profession is held in extremely high confidence by the public at large.

An ethical dilemma occurs when two or more moral obligations or values conflict or compete and the appropriate choice in the situation is unclear. Exercising moral accountablity means the nurse will make a reasoned judgment about what is right and will act accordingly. An individual nurse's determination of what is right may or may not be the same decision that others, including those to whom the nurse is accountable, believe is the right decision. Moral accountability does not mean congruence with others, but rather that nurses will be able adequately to defend and justify their decisions on moral grounds.

Ethical accountability requires decision making on the part of the nurse. Application of an ethical framework or decision-making process to issues of moral concern is helpful to the analysis of an ethical question. Application of a reflective ethical framework to questions about what the nurse should do results not only in decisions that the nurse feels are right or good, but also in actions that can be justified by the nurse. Preferably, ethical analysis by the nurse should not require an emergency situation, but rather thoughtful applications of an ethical framework or decision making process with reflection on values and principles as a means to resolving conflict should be part of a nurse's daily routine. Obviously, in the clinical setting, time is often a luxury; therefore, prior familiarity with ethical theory and a framework for ethical decision makingis essential. For example, making ethical determinations at the time a when treatment is ordered "stat" or staffing decisions must be made are examples of decisions that do not afford the luxury of lengthy deliberation.

Interpretive Statements

The purpose of the interpretive statements related to Provision 4 of the Code of Ethics for Nurses is to develop more fully the meaning of accountability and responsibility in nursing practice in order to provide consistent, universal application of the provision's intent. The interpretive statements provide nurses with a social context for application of the provisions in practice and help to define them within the expanded roles of the nursing profession.

Practical Application of Interpretive Statements

Acceptance of Accountability and Responsibility

Accountability is both related to answerability and responsibility. Accountability is judgment and action on the part of the nurse for which the nurse is answerable to self and others for those judgments and actions. Responsibility refers to the specific accountability or liability associated with the performance of duties of a particular nursing role and may, at times be shared in the sense that a portion of responsibility may be seen as belonging to another who was involved in the situation. Nursing practice is individualized and the responsibilities of the nurse are role dependent. The individual role of the nurse carries with it specific duties and obligations. To meet the role obligations of the nursing profession, the nurse must be familiar with the scope and standards of the profession as well as those of the specific role carried out by the nurse. Regardless of nursing role, the nurse must adhere to the scope and standards of practice when performing or assigning the duties within that role in order to ensure safe, high-quality patient care. Depending on the role of the nurse, the standards are layered and become more complicated as the expertise, complexity, and expectations of that role increases.

Nurses are expected to be able to justify actions based upon nursing skill and knowledge and the application of the nursing process, critical thinking, and nursing knowledge to the care they provide. For example, at a novice or entry level, a professional nurse would have: an understanding of the current scope and standards of practice, the Code of Ethics, and Nursing's Social Policy Statement; the basic knowledge and skills needed to demonstrate competency in the practice of nursing and a working knowledge of the laws and policies that govern nursing practice. Thus, a newly licensed nurse would not be expected to be able to make a decision about whether the healthcare organization in which they worked had acted appropriately or had instead put nurses and patients at risk when a management decision was made to pull a nurse from direct care for other nonpatient care-related duties. Conversely, nurses who choose to develop expertise or to specialize would add to the basic level of their understanding advanced knowledge and skill defined by the nursing literature and specific specialty standards and guidelines that extend beyond the level defined for generic entry into the nursing profession. Thus, a nurse manager or senior level nursing administrator would be expected to be able to evaluate whether the removal of a nurse from staffing was a right or wrong decision.

Instilling professional nursing accountability into direct or indirect patient care helps to ensure accurate, safe, high quality service. The nurse is held accountable for making adjustments to practice based upon changing systems of care. Technology, medicine, and health care are constantly changing, and so must the nurse's knowledge and practice change with the environment. When practice changes occur the nurse may need to seek education and consultation prior to accepting responsibilities. Ultimately, nurses carry out their duties or assign activities to others using nursing knowledge and judgment to assess, evaluate, and determine the appropriate course of action. Even where tasks are assigned to others, the nurse who delegates or assigns these retains accountability and responsibility for those them; this is to say, that tasks and activities can be delegated or assigned, but duties cannot.

Accountability for Nursing Judgment and Action

Accountability for nursing judgment and action means that nurses act under a code of ethical conduct that is grounded in moral principles of fidelity (faithfulness) and respect for dignity, worth, and self-determination of patients. Interpretive statement 4.2 makes clear that accountability and responsibility for nursing practice are an extension of the first three provisions of the Code of Ethics for Nurses which relate to the fundamental values and commitments of the nurse. At every point of practice, from novice to expert practitioner, the nurse is expected to bear responsibility for the care provided and the practice activities (both direct and indirect) irrespective of the particular role the nurse is fulfilling. The moral standard of the profession is one to which nurses must hold themselves and their peers in order to be held accountable in for their practice.

In order to avoid moral conflict or distress, the nurse must uphold personal values and belief systems, regardless of the organizational policies and procedures. If a nurse becomes aware of a conflict between a personal belief and an organizational policy, the nurse must rely on nursing values and practice standards to strive for a higher level of accountability (Hook and White, 2003). Some decisions related to making choices in nursing practice where there are conflicts between nurses and the organization may result in consequences to the nurses including but not limited to reprimand and dismissal. Individual accountability and responsibility for practice may require nurses to choose what they believe is the right and just path even though that choice may not be what the organization or employer desires from them.

Consider situations where nurses finds themseves at odds with the policies of the healthcare organization. A nurse working in a newborn nursery discovers that the mother of a newborn infant admits to using cocaine frequently prior to the child's birth. The nurse believes it is in the best interest of the baby to test the baby for cocaine. The healthcare organization's policy is that no laboratory tests can be performed on a newborn without the express order of the attending physician. The nurse contacts the attending physician who refuses to order the blood test because in his words he "doesn't want to waste his time dealing with the bureaucracy." The nurse is concerned for the baby's welfare and knows that the baby will likely be discharged with the mother later in the day with no follow-up care. The nurse also knows that the State Department of Child Welfare will not attend to the situation unless the infant has a positive drug screen on record. The nurse's supervisor believes the situation to be a matter of judgment and that it is within the physician's prerogative to refuse to order the test. The supervisor suggests that the nurse give up any attempts to convince the physician.

The nurse may find that an effort to protect and advocate for the newborn may carry the risk of being considered insubordinate. Does the accountability for nursing judgment and action change in this case when the nurse is a student reading the chart in preparation for a clinical assignment, when the nurse is experienced, or when the nurse is the supervisor in this case? Consider further the consequences of moral action if the physician reports the nurse for the unlawful practice of medicine because of informing the child's grandparent that a specific request should be made for a drug screen prior to the infant's discharge in order to ascertain what care and treatment the child will be needed. Contrast the nurse's risks against the risk to the child's health assuming the newborn has a sufficient blood level that would indicate symptoms of withdrawal. Does the risk change if the infant begins to suffer withdrawal from the narcotic without care or proper treatment? In this situation and others, the nurse may find it necessary to act on behalf of the patient even though the consequences might put them at personal risk. Consultation by the nurse with the institution's ethics committee may be an appropriate course of action if sufficient time and committee resources are available to assist in deliberation on this dilemma.

Responsibility for Nursing Judgment and Action

Universal recognition of the significance of individual accountability or liability for the duties inherent in the nursing role validates nursing as a profession. With the recognition of nursing as a profession comes the additional responsibility for nurses individually to self-assess for competence. Attached to assessment is the responsibility to seek consultation and continuing education where the nurse finds a lack of knowledge on any pertinent subject. Being responsible for nursing judgments and actions implies that the nurse is answerable for nursing action associated with the duties of a particular role. Being answerable individually for one's nursing knowledge and actions increases the respect and autonomy sought by nurses both from the public and within the arena of healthcare professionals. Embodied in public respect is the need for nurses to be competent in their care. Competence implies continued self-assessment of nursing abilities and the quest to update skills, including those of a technical nature. Self-assessment is the continued review of competence related to nursing judgments, including decisions to delegate nursing activities or tasks (Curtis, 2004).

Liability occurs when the nurse breaches a duty or obligation associated with the performance of a particular nursing role. Legal liability can take several forms. The legal action can be administrative as in a licensure proceeding; civil as in a malpractice action; criminal if the conduct of the nurse is defined in criminal law; or employment related. Legal liability stems from violations of the law and breaches of legal duty, and not necessarily from moral or ethical obligations.

Often, the law and ethics overlap, especially in areas of health care such as dying, privacy and confidentiality, and human rights. Ideally, the legal system would follow ethical thinking and consensus. Unfortunately, what is ethical may not be either covered in law or inadequately covered in law. In fact, some laws may actually be unethical. The law is useful as a consideration of fact and precedent for ethical decision making; however, laws do not direct or control nursing ethics or morals. The Code of Ethics for Nurses is a statement of moral obligations and duties intended to guide the practice of nursing; it is not a legal document.

The following example illustrates competence: A junior nursing instructor, Ida, with two years of teaching experience is responsible for overseeing a group of students during their clinical rotation. Previously, Ida had nine clinical students in a clinical group. One of Ida's prior students made a serious medication error when she ignored and violated a school policy that required approval of the instructor prior to the administration of medication. The school and the hospital are still investigating the incident and the student has been suspended pending further investigation and action by the admission and progression committee.

Ida is vaguely aware of a state board of nursing ruling limiting clinical groups to 10 students, but believes she must be mistaken since her chair has assigned her 12 students. Although, intimidated by her chairperson, Ida makes a weak request for support for teaching such a large group. When chastised by the chair, the instructor withdrawals her request for faculty support. The 12 new students are placed on an adult medicine unit for their clinical. Students in prior groups rated the unit as an excellent unit for student learning. Ida, anxious about her potential liability, makes a conscious decision that the students will have inadequate experience to perform assessments and assist the patients with activities of daily living. Ida does not believe the students can be adequately supervised; therefore, she determines most clinical experiences will only be observational. Other clinical experiences indicated in the syllabus include administering medications, charting, and nursing treatment procedures. The students pass the clinical rotation with excellent grades and enter their second year of nursing school unprepared to move into the junior-level objectives having had only observational clinical experiences without actual supervised practice.

Has Ida, the nursing instructor, neglected her responsibility in providing appropriate clinical experience and skills to the students? The nursing instructor has failed to assess self-competence and seek appropriate resources for herself. In addition, the instructor has failed to properly utilize the learning resources. The actions of a prior student to disregard academic policy would not impact the accountability of the instructor's nursing judgment and accountability since the student's act was self-chosen and against a school policy that was communicated in class and in the syllabus. The student willfully violated the policy in an inappropriate exercise of autonomy. A nursing student who freely and deliberately chooses with full knowledge to act in a manner that directly violates school policy would be individually accountable and responsible for the consequences of those actions.

In the scenario, the school administrator should be held accountable for failing to meet the responsibility of the administrator role. The administrator is responsible to hire and support qualified instructors. Newly hired faculty should be given appropriate support, mentoring, and resources to carry out clinical teaching requirements. The administrator must provide support for the instructor or, in the alternative, relieve the instructor of clinical instruction duties if the instructor is not clinically competent to carry out those duties necessary to help the class achieve completion of the mandatory skills set forth in the curriculum. If the administrator is acting in a manner prohibited by law in assigning a ratio of 1:12 rather than the legally mandated 1:10 or less, then obviously that administrator is acting in an irresponsible matter that could lead to legal liability related to role performance, and is in violation of the expectations of the code for administrative accountability and responsibility.

Delegation of Nursing Activities

Nurses must accept accountability for patient care even when they direct or delegate activities and tasks to others. The ANA defines delegation as "transferring the responsibility for the performance of an activity from one person to another while retaining accountability for the outcome" (ANA, 1995). Delegation generally involves the assignment of activities or tasks related to patient care to less skilled healthcare workers. The registered nurse cannot delegate responsibilities related to making nursing judgments except to another qualified registered nurse. Examples of nursing activities that cannot be delegated to less skilled healthcare workers include but are not limited to assessment and evaluation of the impact of interventions on care provided to the patient.

Delegation can significantly impact the quality of care since many healthcare facilities require a team approach to nursing and do not support a nurse working independently as the sole provider of care. This is to say that social and institutional factors may make the moral dimensions of accountability and responsibility in delegation particularly challenging. Delegation of nursing activities require the nurse to consider not only the tasks at hand, but also the ability and competence of those to whom the tasks are assigned. Effective delegation can increase productivity because it allows staff of varying skill levels to succeed in doing a few smaller tasks well rather than multiple tasks poorly (Quallich, 2005). Assignment or delegation does not mean the nurse is giving up accountability or responsibility. The nurse is still accountable for any decision to delegate activities and remains responsible for supervising or monitoring those to whom tasks were delegated. Accountability exists not only in what the nurse can or cannot delegate, but also in knowing what tasks or activities other less skilled healthcare workers on the team are capable of doing. Employer policies or directives that state what activities a person is competent to do within a job classification are not sufficient to relieve the nurse of responsibility for making independent judgments about delegation and assignment of nursing tasks. The complexity of delegating nursing tasks has prompted the development of many models of delegation that appear in both the literature and state nursing regulations across the country.

Nurses who function as managers or administrators have a particular responsibility to facilitate appropriate assignments and delegation. This is sometimes complicated by difficult institutional policies around staffing, and can be compounded by a nursing shortage. The role of the manager or charge nurse, past and present, takes on one of the highest levels of delegation in the nursing profession. Nightingale in *Notes on Nursing* (1869) states that being in charge is not just about doing nursing tasks by oneself or appointing tasks to others, but also includes ensuring that others complete the duties to which they were appointed.

The difficulty of making determinations related to delegation can be demonstrated in the following example. Nancy, a registered professional nurse, has a six-patient assignment on a busy inpatient medical/surgical unit on the day shift. Nancy's unit is short a clinical associate; however, Nancy is fortunate to be assigned a clinical associate from the outpatient neurology unit. About halfway through the shift, Nancy discharges one patient from the unit. Shortly after the discharge, she is notified by the admission clerk that a new patient will be admitted to the empty bed. While Nancy is doing her assessment on the newly admitted patient, she is notified by the clinical associate of a greater than one degree Celsius elevation in temperature of a patient receiving a blood transfusion.

The patient receiving the transfusion is a middle-aged male surgical patient receiving his second unit of blood due to a postoperative hemoglobin of 7.0mg/dl following a total hip replacement. The first unit of blood was tolerated without incident. The new admission is an elderly female with a complicated past medical history with an elbow fracture as the result of a fall. The patient was admitted through the emergency room following an ambulance transport. The new admission is complaining of pain "all over" and is requiring an extended period of Nancy's time in order to complete the assessment and admission process. Nancy asks the clinical associate to recheck the male patient and make a determination whether or not the charge nurse should be given the information regarding the patient receiving the transfusion and the elevated temperature.

Upon completing the admission process and administering pain medication to the new admission, Nancy returns to the nurse's station to record a report for the oncoming afternoon shift. After Nancy finishes her report, she is informed that the family of the newly admitted patient has arrived and is requesting to speak with the patient's nurse about the plan of care. Nancy returns to the new patient's room to speak with the family and fails to follow up on the febrile patient.

This situation raises questions about appropriate delegation of care. Has the nurse appropriately transferred responsibility and accountability for the febrile patient to another person? Can the nurse expect the clinical associate to make a determination regarding the patient and the necessity of informing the charge nurse so that perhaps some action could be taken related to the care of the patient receiving the blood transfusion? Obviously, the nurse would be responsible for the judgment she made to continue with her assessment of the new admission versus taking an action that would provide the patient who has demonstrated the potential for a blood reaction with appropriate nursing care. The attempt to delegate the responsibility to a clinical associate is unacceptable since only a task and not a judgment can be delegated to a less skilled healthcare worker. Perhaps the scenario will be resolved as the nurse intended and the charge nurse would assume responsibility for the assessment and care of the febrile patient. However, Nancy did not act to assure that this would happen if the rise in temperature did not, in fact, signal a transfusion reaction. Consider the consequences if the scenario does not go as the Nancy intended and the febrile patient is not provided care until the nurse completes her discussion with the newly admitted patient's family. What if the condition of the febrile patient worsens? What if the reaction to the blood is severe resulting in shock and even death? The need to attend to a potential transfusion reaction greatly outweighs a need to finish an assessment and admission. What options could or should Nancy have considered with regard to the patient receiving the transfusion or the patient being admitted?

Case Example

The Manager with Insufficient Staff

Susan, a nurse manager for a busy adult trauma unit, is facing staffing shortages for the upcoming schedule. Susan cannot cover all three shifts with a complement of two nurses. Susan knows that if she does not have two nurses per shift that the RN on duty would not be able to leave the unit and that the nurse may not get a break from nursing responsibilities over the course of the 8-hour shift. No new applications for employment have been received by the manager by the time the schedule is due to be posted. Susan is aware that even with new hires, there will be a delay in fulfilling the staffing needs due to the orientation process that all new hires are required to attend. The unit previously functioned using an established staffing pattern based on the acuity of the patients. Susan has voiced concerns to the Vice President of Nursing and Allied Services over the lack of staff, but is given no immediate solutions and told to deal with it. Seeing no alternative to the impending crisis, the manager institutes a change in staffing patterns without notifying the staff. The patient to staff ratio will be significantly increased and, at night, the RN will be the sole nurse on the unit without relief. Nurses will rotate the night shift. Following two serious incidents on the night shift, a staff nurse anonymously reports Susan's actions as unsafe practice to the State Board of Nursing. As a result of the impending investigation by the Board, Susan talks to the hospital licensing facility and the local newspaper about the staffing situation at the hospital. Consequently, the hospital receives bad press and is contacted by the hospital licensing authority. As a result, Susan is fired. ■

What options were available to Susan when she was told to "deal with it" in being short-staffed? Who is accountable and responsible for the rise in incidents on the night shift? Was it appropriate for the staff nurse to report Susan to the Board? Was it appropriate for Susan to talk to the hospital licensing organization and the local newspaper? Was Susan's firing appropriate?

Summary

The commitment to the nursing profession starts with a strong and clear understanding of the ethical code of conduct, including responsibility and accountability for individual nursing practice. If nurses are not held accountable for their actions, nursing can not be considered a profession. The nurse's obligation to provide optimal patient care is often challenged by limited resources and a strained healthcare system. The Code of Ethics for Nurses demands that nurses practice in a responsible and ethical manner. As recognized first by Florence Nightingale and today by our society, the prestige of the profession of nursing depends on a universal commitment to accountability and responsibility. As depicted in the case study examples, accountability issues may arise at any level or role within the nursing profession. The nurse must always be aware of the potential outcome in any given situation and be willing to take responsibility for individual actions and knowledge. Regardless of the role held within the nursing profession, accountability for all aspects of individual nursing practice leads to the successful completion of the nurse's obligation to provide optimum patient care (ANA, 2001).

References

All online references were accessed in December 2007.

American Nurses Association. 2001. *Code of Ethics for Nurses with Interpretive Statements*. Washington, DC: American Nurses Publishing.

American Nurses Association. 1995. Position statements: Registered nurse utilization of unlicensed assistive personnel. Washington, DC: ANA. http://www.nursingworld.org/ readroom/position/uap/uapuse.htm.

Burkhart, M.A., and A.K. Nathaniel. 2002. *Ethics and Issues in Contemporary Nursing*, 2nd ed. Albany, NY: Delmar.

Curtis, E., and H. Nicholl. 2004. Delegation: A key function of nursing. *Nursing Management* 11(4): 26–31.

Gallup Poll (December 14, 2006). Nurses top list of most honest and ethical professions. http://www.galluppoll.com/content/?ci=25888&pg=1.

Hook, K.G., and G.B. White. 2003. *Code of Ethics for Nurses with Interpretive Statements: An independent study module*. Washington, DC: ANA. http://www.nursingworld.org/ mods/mod580/cecdefull.htm.

Nightingale, F. 1869. *Notes on Nursing: What It Is, And What It Is Not*. New York: Dover Publications.

Quallich, S.A. 2005. A bond of trust: Delegation. *Urologic Nursing* 25(2): 120–23.

About the Author

Laurie A. Badzek, JD, LLM, MS, RN, NAP, is currently Director of the American Nurses Association Center of Ethics and Human Rights, a role in which she previously served from 1998–99. During that time, Badzek was instrumental in developing a plan that ultimately resulted in the approval of a new Code of Ethics for Nurses by the 2001 House of Delegates. Currently a tenured, full professor at the West Virginia University School of Nursing, Badzek, a nurse attorney, teaches nursing, ethics, law, and health policy. Having practiced in a variety of nursing and law positions, she is an active researcher, investigating ethical and legal healthcare issues. Her current research interests include patient and family decision making, nutraceutical use, mature minors, genomics, and professional healthcare ethics. Her research has been published in nursing, medical, and communication studies journals, including *Journal of Nursing Law, Nephrology Nursing Journal, Annals of Internal Medicine, Journal of Palliative Care,* and *Health Communication.*

Provision
Five

The nurse owes the same duties to self as to others,
including the responsibility to preserve integrity and safety,
to maintain competence, and to continue personal and
professional growth.

Provision Five

Marsha D.M. Fowler, PhD, MDiv, MS, RN, FAAN

The Suggested Code of 1926 states that "the most precious possession of this profession is the ideal of service, extending even to the sacrifice of life itself."[1] This somewhat overwrought statement does correctly identify the central moral motif of the profession: the ideal of service. And yet, it also presents us with one of the central tensions of the profession, that of serving over against extending one's self too far or of risking harm to self. Need service extend even to the sacrifice of life itself? On the absolutely practical side, this would be a serious hindrance for nurse recruiters! Setting aside extraordinary circumstances under which nurses might chose to risk their lives, nurses do have a duty to tend to their own well-being, not to place themselves in harm's way, or, as the provision asserts, nurses have duties to self that ought to be observed.[2] The principle of duties to self (sometimes called "the principle of self-regarding duties") can be divided into four main features: a duty of moral self-respect, a duty of professional growth and maintenance of competence, a duty of maintaining wholeness of character, and a duty of the preservation of one's integrity. These are collectively understood as a single duty of "duties to self."

Duties to Self

The first and only substantive work on the obligation of duties to self in the nursing literature is Andrew Jameton's essay "Duties to self: Professional Nursing in the Critical Care Unit."[3] Jameton notes that some philosophers, such as John Stuart Mill, have denied "that it is meaningful to talk of duties to self," but that others, including Aquinas, Kant, and Hume, "assert the meaningfulness of speaking of duties to oneself."[4] The arguments against a notion of duties to self center on our inability to enforce such duties, specifically, that it is not meaningful to speak of self-coercion and, secondly, that we cannot release ourselves from such duties. Arguments for a notion of duties to self emphasize that while I cannot force myself to meet such a duty, even so, I am answerable for not meeting them and that duties to self are an instrumental good, that is, a good that serves to support my duties to others. Note that duties to self differ from self-centeredness or entitlement in that they specifically support my moral duties to others. The strongest argument for a notion of duties to self resides in the concept of universal obligations. If an obligation applies to everyone, then I am not exempt from the collective "everyone," and those duties apply to myself as well. Immanuel Kant's second formulation of the categorical imperative (his rule for moral rule-making) makes clear the inclusion of one's self in the universal: "Act so that you treat humanity, *whether in your own person* or in that of another, always as an end and never as a means" [italics added].[5]

The nursing ethics literature from the 1800s to the present has affirmed an obligation of duties to self. One of the earliest such references is found in *Trained Nurse and Hospital Review*, July 1889. The article by "H.C.C." (an otherwise unidentified superintendent of a training school in Boston), is entitled "Ethics in nursing: A nurse's duties to herself: Talks of a superintendent with her graduating class."[6] The focus of the article is on rest and bodily care as essential to the health of the nurse for the sake of the ability to meet her duties to patients. (In that period, nurses were exclusively female.) Particular concern is directed toward the dedicated, energetic nurse who may overextend and risk personal health in the course of care-giving. H.C.C. writes: "Please remember I am only speaking to the good nurses—the enthusiastic one—poor nurses, lazy nurses, have no temptation to overwork themselves. They may die of indigestion but they will not die of exhaustion."[7] Many of the early nursing ethics books echoed an emphasis upon duties to self. Isabel Robb's oft reprinted *Nursing Ethics: For Hospital and Private Use* (1900) places considerable emphasis on a range of duties to self.[8]

This emphasis on self-regarding duties has for decades remained prominent in nursing ethics literature, including the earliest codes. The Tentative Code of 1940, one of the early unadopted codes for nursing, includes a section on the nurse's responsibilities to herself. It states: "A nurse is to keep herself physically, mentally, and morally fit, and to provide for spiritual, intellectual, and professional growth. She should institute savings plans which will bring her financial security in her old age."[9] While the emphasis on duties to self persists in the nursing literature, especially in textbooks, it departs from the later codes. The incorporation of a provision on self-regarding duties in the present code is indeed a "reappearance" rather than something "new."

Interpretive Statement 5.1: Moral Self-Respect

This section introduces this duty and grounds it in the self-inclusiveness of universal duties: what I owe to others as moral duties, I likewise owe to myself as a moral duty. Without so stating, this would mean that all of the provisions that apply to patients would also apply to oneself. For instance, Provision 1 states that "the nurse, in all professional relationships practices with compassion and respect for the inherent dignity, worth, and uniqueness of every individual."[10] Self-respect, then, becomes one of the many duties owed oneself.

The focus of the interpretive statement is on explaining the several distinguishably different areas of concern. Jameton has identified three such aspects of duties to self: *integrity, self-regarding duties,* and *identity. Identity* refers to the coherent integration of one's personal and professional identity—what I am morally as a person, I am morally as a nurse. According to Jameton, identity includes concerns for maintaining ideals, the meaningfulness of work, expression of one's opinion, concern for wrongs committed by others, and participation in moral judgment in the work setting. *Self-regarding duties* refers to "duties [that] have a content that affects or applies to oneself primarily," here *competence* is of specific concern. *Integrity* includes wholeness of character, attention to one's own welfare or self-care, and emotional integrity reliant upon maintaining relational boundaries.[11] The current provision is indebted to Jameton for his pioneering work, and incorporates his three aspects in three somewhat different divisions: *professional growth and maintenance of competence, wholeness of character,* and *preservation of integrity.*

Interpretive Statement 5.2: Professional Growth and Maintenance of Competence

Previous codes, such as the Suggested Code of 1926 and the Tentative Code of 1940, have included a responsibility for ongoing professional growth. The Suggested Code states:

Professional growth and development are promoted by membership in professional organizations, both state and local, by attendance at meetings and conventions and by constant reading on professional subjects. Yet further growth may be assured by attendance on institutes and postgraduate courses.[12]

Though the context is that of professional growth as a duty to self, it does not so much discuss professional growth as it does how one might go about growing professionally.

The Tentative Code of 1940 is not quite so specific; it declares a "requirement of continuous study and growth" and a duty for the nurse "to provide for spiritual, intellectual and professional growth," as noted above.[13] In several codes, such as that of 1950, the nurse is responsible for "continued reading, study, observation, and investigation," not strictly as a duty to self, but rather as a duty to the profession in order that the social/professional status of nursing, and the status of the individual nurse as a professional, may be maintained.[14] Notice, however, that it moves beyond continued study and reading for self-development, or even to better serve the patient; instead, it casts the duty in terms of maintaining the stature of nursing as a profession, as well as the social prestige of nursing. Nursing has, of course, struggled for years for the social recognition accorded professions. The Tentative Code even opens with the assertion "Nursing is a profession," and then goes on to defend that assertion with a sizable amount of material that is not actually appropriate to a code of ethics.[15] Here, the concern is for the profession and its professionalism, not for the nurse, so it could be argued that, in this particular statement formulation, it may not be a duty to self.

The emphasis upon professional growth as a duty to self shifted over the years in two ways. First, it shifted from a duty to self to a duty to the profession for the sake of the profession. Second, it shifted in the direction of an increasing concern for competence, not only for the sake of the profession, but also for that of the patient as well. Though they have been used as if interchangeable, "professional growth" and "competence" are not the same. Competence is the rock bottom level of acceptable practice, the level below which no practitioner should fall. Professional growth moves the nurse beyond mere competence, as a minimum standard of practice, toward excellence and is thus directed toward an ideal of practice. The Code of 1985 merges professional growth and competence and their ends, stating that:

> For the client's optimum well-being and for the nurses' own professional development, the care of the client reflects and incorporates new techniques and knowledge in health care as these develop, especially as they relate to the nurse's particular field of practice. The nurse must be aware of the need for continued professional learning and must assume personal responsibility for currency of knowledge and skills.[16]

Though the Codes have presented professional growth as necessary to competence for the sake of the profession's stature and for the welfare of the recipient of nursing care, Jameton argues that competence is instead a self-regarding duty, primarily directed toward oneself. He writes:

> Competence is...primarily...an attribute of self to be cultivated, and secondarily as a means of affecting patients.... Nursing, as a practice, provides a set of "internal" goods that are satisfying in themselves. Internal goods are the intrinsic excellences of good nursing practice, as distinguished from external rewards such as salary, the gratitude of patients, and so forth. The existence

of intrinsic conceptions or excellence makes it possible for nurses to regard development of competence as a matter of self-development rather than simply a matter of achieving external rewards through affecting others.[17]

Without denying that competence affects others, this new Code of Ethics more clearly and vigorously casts competence as a self-regarding duty, essential to self-respect and self-esteem, professional status, and the meaningfulness of work. It ties professional growth to a commitment to life-long learning reminiscent of the early nursing ethics literature. Professional growth is not limited to the knowledge and skill necessary for patient care, but also includes "issues, concerns, controversies, and ethics."[18]

The emphasis upon competence, per se, was given even more emphasis in the 1960 Code for Professional Nurses and succeeding codes. Provision 8 of that 1960 Code states: "The nurse maintains professional competence and demonstrates concern for the competence of other members of the nursing profession."[19] Over the next several decades, competence as articulated in the Codes takes four emphases: the professional competence of the nurse; the competent nurse forced by circumstances (e.g., staff reductions) to practice less competently; the duty to act upon observed incompetence of nurses, physicians, or others; and the duty to delegate tasks only in accord with the competence of others. Only the first and second of these refers to a self-regarding duty of competence. As a self-regarding duty, the Code of 2001 calls for ongoing and authentic self-evaluation and peer review as a means of evaluating one's performance.

Interpretive Statement 5.3: Wholeness of Character

Can a person who is a rogue, scoundrel, liar, and cheat in personal life be a virtuous nurse in professional life? It is unlikely. What we are personally, we are professionally. Our personal and professional identities are neither separate, nor coextensive; they are integrated and deeply commingled, mutually influencing each other. The person who has become "a nurse," as opposed to the person who "does nursing," is one who has incorporated and integrated the values of the profession with personal values. The Suggested Code of 1926 notes that "the nurse who fails to find happiness in her work is not truly a nurse."[20] Persons who do not find happiness in their work have always been of special concern to nursing educators. It is unfortunate that some nursing students are misplaced in nursing, finding little congruence with the values of the profession, and having insufficient personal insight to see the conflict between their personal identity and their budding professional identity. Indeed, some students never fully become nurses; in fact, some are alienated toward nursing, and yet they can develop the knowledge and skill to complete a nursing education with considerable success and to pass the Board exams with flying colors.

Case Example 1

Consider the quandary of Prof. Svetlana Scythe. Senior student Allison Baxter has enrolled in Prof. Scythe's Nursing Issues and Trends class and Community Health clinical lab. Allison has a GPA of 3.8, is technically proficient in clinical practice, has reasonable communication and interpersonal skills in patient care, is able to prioritize and manage a patient load, and is generally quite capable in nursing theory and practice. But, she hates nursing. She had wanted to be a paramedic with the fire department, but could not get in because of the exceptionally competitive applications and the very long waiting list. In the end, her father pushed her into nursing school. For all her ability, she does not identify with nursing, nor does she want to and, indeed, in discussions in the Issues and Trends class, as well as in the Community Health course, has an "attitude" toward nursing and speaks ill of the profession among her friends.

Prof. Scythe, as well as other faculty members over the years have tried to counsel Ms. Baxter as to whether she should consider leaving the school, but she will not consider leaving, in part because of parental pressure, in part because she did not want to "start all over" in school, and because it would shortly afford her an acceptable income. In its student handbook, the school affirms the ANA Code of Ethics as one of their standards of practice. In many ways, the Code enjoins nurses to work for the welfare and advance of the profession. The faculty are very concerned about graduating this student, but can they refuse to graduate a student who has an excellent academic record, but who has an anti-nursing attitude and does not embrace the values of nursing, based on a generic school affirmation of the Code? Unfortunately no. ■

Laws only demand that they be obeyed, and not that one be a good person besides. Ethics, of course, demand that we be good persons, beyond the expectations of "requirements." The Code of 1985 states:

> Nursing is responsible and accountable for admitting to the profession only those individuals who have demonstrated the knowledge, skills, and commitment considered essential for nursing practice. Nurse educators have a major responsibility for ensuring that these competencies and a demonstrated commitment to professional practice have been achieved before entry of an individual into the practice of professional nursing.[21]

Course and program requirements of schools function like the law: you must meet them but they cannot demand that you be a "good nurse" in the sense of affirming nursing and embracing a nursing identity. However, where a student clearly fails to identify with nursing, vigorous and consistent attempts should be made from the earliest point onward to counsel the student to leave the program with the hope of moving them earlier into another more suitable discipline, with less time lost. In addition, faculty can decline to give letters of recommendation if there is no evidence of change. In situations such as this, it is more than likely that the graduate will not find work meaningful, and in fact may come to hate it, and may leave the profession. She or he may also stay in this "bad marriage," but that is a matter of choice.

Not everyone is suited to nursing; admissions criteria and screening should be sufficiently rigorous as to ascertain a student's "fit" with nursing, and postadmission follow-ups and advising must be vigilant to redirect students when necessary. A more intentional and hearty emphasis on embracing the values and ethics of the profession, including the Code, from the earliest courses on would strengthen the curriculum and might serve as a deterrent to those who in the end will not "become nurses" in the moral sense. There is also an important place for courses on nursing history in this endeavor. While the case presents a moral quandary for nursing educators, as the 1985 Code makes evident, it is implied in the language of the Code of 2001 that Allison's failure to come to a congruence between personal and professional identity indicates an unfortunate failure in duties to self and forecasts an unhappy professional future for her.

As an additional example, a similar situation sometimes can occur in nursing in some of the accelerated generic master's degree programs that take in persons with baccalaureates in non-nursing disciplines. Consider the case of Bob, an aerospace engineer with a Master's degree who was laid off in the last defense-contract cycle of lay-offs. He saw a colleague apply to nursing school, asked about entry level salaries, and decided that nursing would be a quick and easy fix to his situation. He entered an accelerated generic program. He easily mastered the essential and technical skills, did exceptionally well academically, and moved very rapidly through the program. However, he did not become socialized into the value structure of the profession. The program, though accelerated, did attend to professional socialization and the values of the program, but Bob did not. He retained the value structure of his prior discipline, rocket science, and consistently remarked that "nursing is not rocket science." His relationship with patients was one of superiority and "hard facts," lacking warmth and compassion. In these days of "outsourcing," not all persons come into nursing with altruistic or pristine motives, nor do they need to. However, in nursing education, it is crucial that attention be given to "formation." Nursing values must be cultivated and inculcated in these adult learners, and integrated into their personal value structure so that they assume a proper nursing identity, if they themselves, the patient, and the profession, are to be well served.

We bring our whole selves to nursing, not just our professional identity. That means that we bring our personal and our professional moral values in one package to the issues, concerns, and dilemmas that confront us in practice. The new Code states that "duties to self involve an authentic expression of one's own moral point-of-view in practice."[22] Sometimes, this moral point of view is more professional than personal, and, other times, more personal than professional in derivation.

Case Example 2

Consider Father Mac James, a patient on dialysis following nephrectomy for renal carcinoma. Because of congenital cysts in his other kidney it was expected that he would have to remain on dialysis for life. At one point he became clinically depressed and was successfully treated with electroconvulsive therapy when medications failed to be effective. At the time, he felt that he wanted to "give up," but also felt an obligation as a retired priest to accept treatment. For two years, despite suffering from postdepression, he continued with dialysis. One day, when the CNS visiting nurse, Abby Davids, saw him, he told her that he wanted to stop dialysis on July 23, following his 40th anniversary as a priest. He said that his quality of life was unacceptable, would not improve, and that he had lived long enough. He said he had "a sense of peace" about his decision. His family was deeply distressed and tried to coerce him into change his mind. After all, "he isn't that old," they said. The physicians started antidepressant medication, but to no effect; he did not change his mind. In the clinical care conference, all parties were agreed that they wanted Father Mac to continue his dialysis, except Abby. She has had several discussions with him and believes that his was a reasoned, reflective position, consistent with his beliefs and values, even if he could live a number of years longer on dialysis. However, at the patient care conference, she felt the full weight of the consensus against her. Should she speak up?

Yes. This does not mean that her view will prevail. This does not mean that they are guaranteed to listen. Even when persons of moral good will come together to discuss life and death issues, there may be disagreement. One does not have a duty to self to express personal values so that others might be persuaded differently. The duty to self is to express one's professional moral point of view, to preserve one's authenticity; in other words, to be true to one's self. In addition, doing so maintains open moral dialogue, which is not achieved if different views are suppressed. In some cases, this moral expression may be the only explicitly nursing moral voice, a voice that might not be heard if the nurse fails to speak up. Sometimes, however, the moral point of view being expressed arises from the nurse's personal values in a professional context. ■

Case Example 3

Consider Michael Tucker, a hospice nurse and a lifelong Evangelical Christian in a largely Jewish facility. For Michael, issues of faith are as much matters of life and death as cancer is. In the hospice setting, Michael has ample opportunity to present his faith to his patients and he is ready to do so, but wonders what is or is not morally appropriate. Stan Grossman is his patient. He was reared without religious influences, but identifies himself as Jewish. He is acutely anxious as he sees his life drawing to a close and is reaching out for "answers." Another patient, Miriam Swartz, also Jewish, who likewise seeks answers, but does not feel "panicked" as Stan does, asks Michael about his faith and if it "works" for him. Sophie Adleman knows that her faith is of support to her as she is dying and wants Michael to pray with her and to call the Bikur Cholim because "the Rabbis teach us that visiting a sick person removes 1/60th of his or her illness" and she figures that she needs "only 48 more visitors to be healed." Michael needs to know if he can speak of his faith to Stan or Marv. Also, is it a violation of his own values to call the Bikur Cholim for Sophie and to pray with her?

Morally, may Michael speak of his own Christian faith with Stan? Probably not. Given Stan's anxious state of mind, it is quite possible that Michael's expression of his own faith would be coercive to him. If Michael judges that Stan is looking for spiritual answers, he should start with the answers closest to Stan's own background. If after adequate exploration, it does not suffice, he can enlarge the discussion if Stan so requests. Michael ought to consider the nature and depth of the conversation and secure a professional chaplain for Stan if warranted and welcome. Vulnerable patients may not be evangelized. Doing so is not an expression of a duty to self to be who one is, rather it is taking unfair advantage of a wounded individual; many religions take a dim view of this. May Michael permissibly respond to Miriam with an expression of his personal faith? Probably yes. Miriam has asked a personal question of Michael and looks for a personal answer. Michael is free authentically to express who he is, even in matters of religious faith—or politics—if asked. Miriam has asked a question inviting a religious response and explanation. Michael may give this freely, yet only in a way that preserves Miriam's freedom.

We bring our whole selves to patient care. Michael is a nurse, but he is also a Christian nurse, and that is who he must be for the patient who inquires of him, and that is who he must be for himself. In some instances, being a member of one religion or another need not be made explicit to be consistent with one's self identity. Many times, the religion can be transparent to the patient, yet it remains the grounding motive for the care of others. What about Sophie? Does Michael jeopardize his faith commitment or values by supporting Sophie's explicitly Jewish religious needs? Can he pray with her and remain authentic? Michael has two kinds of religious commitments: those of his own faith and spirituality, and those of his faith that would extend the faith to others. Sophie is not interested in his faith; she is interested in her own. Given this, Michael does not jeopardize or deny his own Christian identity in supporting Sophie in her religion, even in praying with her. His duty to self in preserving his own wholeness of character is not affected by doing so. Since Sophie is not interested in having Michael extend his faith to her, he may not do so. However, he may be a person of faith with another person of faith, bringing their separate faiths together for Sophie's good. In doing this, Michael does not deny his religious value of extending his faith, rather he affirms that the extension of his faith is for those who choose to receive it. Like information in informed consent, it is to be "offered," not imposed. In not offering it where it is not welcome, Michael does not violate any duty to self. Indeed, by refraining from offering faith where it is not welcome, Michael affirms the freedom that must exist in faith. Michael can call the Bikur Cholim, he can pray with Sophie, and he can refrain from evangelism and remain authentically who he is. Early codes made explicit the demand that nurses respect the religious and other beliefs of the patient. Later codes broadened to include a respect for a large range of personal attributes including religious and cultural values. ∎

While this case focuses on religion as an aspect of "wholeness of character" of the nurse, religion is but one example. Some nurses are not religious; what if the nurse in this case was an atheist? Any strong, enduring commitment that forms a part of who the nurse is as a person plays a role in wholeness. Whether it be politics, vegetarianism/veganism, ecofeminism, pacifism, atheism, agnosticism, or any other strongly held commitment, all are a part of who the nurse is authentically and may be shared, or must be withheld from sharing, on the same sorts of grounds as that of religion: "nurses are generally free to express an informed personal opinion as long as this preserves the voluntariness of the patient and maintains appropriate professional and moral boundaries."[23] The role of the nurse is to assist patients in reflecting on their own values, not those of the nurse.

Patients request other kinds of personal information from nurses as well. Increasingly, patients demonstrate well-developed internet skills in sleuthing health problems and illness treatments. Greater or lesser degrees of discernment of the quality of the information make their way to the nurse in the context of health and illness counseling and patient education. Nurses will be asked about alternative or adjunctive therapies, the orange pill, herbals, therapeutic teas, and a virtually endless range of treatments. So, just what *do* you think about the orange pill? Is the nurse free to offer an opinion?

Nurses have professional "relationships" with patients. If this is not the case, then the patient could just as well ask the question of a computer. But patients do not want a computer, they want a living, breathing human nurse. Nurses are generally free to express their *informed* personal opinion in the face of patient inquiries on matters related to health and illness. In professional relationships, however, the boundaries are professional and must be maintained as such. Patient freedom must also be maintained and expressions of personal professional opinion must preserve the patient's voluntariness. Duties to self demand that nurses be who *they* authentically are and, in turn, that patients are permitted to be, and supported in, who they authentically are.

Interpretive Statement 5.4: Preservation of Integrity

Integrity is an internal quality, differing from honesty, which is interpersonal in nature. Thus, integrity is, primarily, a self-concern and a self-regarding duty. Preservation of integrity as a duty to self requires a lived conformity with the values that one holds dear, both personal and professional. Professional nursing values, while individually held, are shared among nurses, so that a duty to self that is jeopardized in the work setting for one nurse may by circumstances apply to all nurses in that setting.

For much of the history of modern nursing, staffing patterns for "general duty" nursing have posed problems for nurses. In a report on the nursing supply in 1928, Burgess wrote the following:

> General floor duty is often the last resort of the desperate private duty nurse. There are reasons for this. In all too many hospitals the superintendent of nurses is expected to get along with an inadequate number of assistants. The result is that the nurses on floor duty are working under tremendous pressure, and as the number of patients swells above normal it is inevitable that much of the nursing service on the ward will be inadequate and improperly given. Good nurses refuse to work that way... the fact is that general duty [i.e., hospital nursing] is not considered respectable. It is despised not only by the nurses themselves but by the hospital authorities. Some hospitals

Guide to the Code of Ethics for Nurses

actually pay the servants and maids and orderlies on their wards as much as they pay graduate nurses.[24]

Too many patients, inadequate number of assistants, overworked nurses, too much pressure—a description from the 1920s that sounds remarkably contemporary! The Code of 1985 makes clear the responsibility of nurses and the nursing profession to participate (individually and collectively) in establishing "conditions of employment that (a) enable the nurse to practice in accordance with the standards of nursing practice and (b) provide a care environment that meets the standards of nursing service."[25] The concern in Provisions 9 and 10 of the 1985 Code are for the preservation of the integrity of nursing. The Code of 2001 furthers these concerns by applying them to the preservation of the integrity of nurses, especially those placed in an economically constrained environment that pressure nurses to practice in ways that violate their professional integrity. Like the Tentative Code, this new code overtly recognizes the moral threats posed by economic constraints in the practice setting, an observation that is lacking in the 1985 Code, as well as earlier versions.

The Code of 2001 also introduces two concepts that are relatively new: that of integrity-preserving compromise and "conscientious objection." In raising the notion of integrity-preserving compromise, the new Code recognizes the competing values that confront nurses, and acknowledging that their values might not prevail. However, nurses need not bow to all other values. Nursing values are to be preserved and nurses are expected to negotiate compromises that will in fact preserve them. This requires, of course, a "community of moral discourse," where nurses speak up and one profession's values do not trump those of others.

The second recent concept is not actually new, but rather involves the introduction of new terminology. "Conscientious objection" is most frequently applied to the refusal on moral or religious grounds to bear arms or to go to war. Prior to the American Revolution, conscientious objectors in this country often came from "pacifist" churches such as the Quakers, Mennonites, and Brethren. As a consequence, these churches have a long tradition of scholarly literature on conscientious objection. When not applied to war or to bearing arms, conscientious objection refers to the moral or religiously based refusal to participate in an activity otherwise required, perhaps even by the law. Thus, in nursing, conscientious objection would be the refusal to participate in some aspect of patient care on moral or religious grounds. This refusal might be based on a moral or religious objection to a specific intervention categorically (e.g., abortion), or moral objection to a particular intervention with a specific patient (as in requiring Father James above to continue dialysis), or a moral objection to a pattern of behavior (e.g., habitual short staffing that forces substandard nursing practice that endangers patient well-being).

Conscientious objection, whether expressed individually or collectively, always involves the refusal to violate a deeply held moral value, personal or professional. Previous codes have always provided a "moral way out" for nurses who were confronted with any one of the three examples noted above. Previous Code specified that, where there is a categorical objection to a particular intervention (e.g., abortion), such objection should be made at the time of employment and that, in no case, should the nurse abandon the patient. This new Code enlarges the discussion, gives it a conceptual framework in conscientious objection, and rightly expresses it as an aspect of duties to self. It also notes that conscientious objection does not insulate a nurse against consequences for having refused to participate in an aspect of nursing practice or patient care.

The benefit of clearly identifying a doctrine of conscientious objection is that it gives nurses a way to conceptualize and articulate a "refusal to care," more accurately a "refusal to participate" in a specific aspect of patient care. In the days before advance directives, when patients were, in hospital parlance, "full code" because a do-not-resuscitate order was not written when it should have been (e.g., no statistical chance of success, or the patient did not want it), nurses might badger the physician to write one, only to encounter foot-dragging. When the patient went into cardiac arrest, some nurses felt the only way out of the dilemma was to engage in a "slow code." Conscientious objection provides a way out of this bind by affording the nurse an opportunity to make a strenuous objection known on moral grounds, and then to make it stick. In other words, conscientious objection permits nurses to preserve their integrity in the face of a clinical activity or situation to which they have moral objections to participation.

Conclusion

Nursing has historically maintained that the nurse owes the same duties to self as to others. In this provision, the new Code reintroduces a concern for duties to self that have always been of historical importance, but had receded from our gaze. However, unlike early discussions of duties to self that focused on the physical health of the nurse, continued education, and savings for old age, this more contemporary aspect of the Code directly extends the discussion into areas of wholeness of character, identity, and integrity not seen in the earlier literature. It recasts competence as a self-regarding duty and not simply as an instrumental good in service to others. Indeed, this provision focuses on the full range of duties to self as nurse-focused, rather than profession- or patient-focused. At first glance, this provision might seem an innovation. Not so. It is something old, something renewed, something borrowed from history, and something true.

Endnotes

1   American Nurses Association. 1926. A suggested code. *American Journal of Nursing* 26(8): 599–601. (For a fuller discussion of the obligation or option to care in the face of risk to the nurse, consult the reference in the next endnote.)

2. American Nurses Association. 2006. *Risk and Responsibility in Providing Nursing Care.* Silver Spring, MD: ANA.

3. Jameton, Andrew. 1985. Duties to self: Professional nursing in the critical care unit. In *Ethics at the Bedside,* Marsha Fowler and June Levine-Ariff, eds., pp. 115–135. Philadelphia: JB Lippincott.

4. Ibid, pp. 117–18.

5. Kant, Immanuel. 1998. *Groundwork of the Metaphysics of Morals,* Mary J. Gregor, ed. Cambridge, England: Cambridge University Press.

6. H.C.C. 1889. Ethics in nursing: A nurse's duty to herself: Talks of a superintendent with her graduating class. *Trained Nurse and Hospital Review* 3(1: July): 1–5.

7. Ibid. Not paginated.

8. Robb, Isabel Adams Hampton. 1900. *Nursing Ethics: For Hospital and Private Use.* New York: E.C. Koeckert.

9. American Nurses Association. 1940. A Tentative Code. *American Journal of Nursing* 40(9): 980.

10. American Nurses Association. 2001. *Code of Ethics for Nurses with Interpretive Statements,* pp. 18–20. Washington, DC: ANA.

11. Jameton. Duties to self, pp. 120–32.

12. American Nurses Association. 1926. A Suggested Code, p. 600.

13. American Nurses Association. 1940. A Tentative Code, pp. 977, 980.

14. American Nurses Association. 1950. *The Code for Professional Nurses*. New York: ANA.

15. American Nurses Association. 1940. A Tentative Code, pp. 977–78.

16. American Nurses Association. 1985. *Code for Nurses with Interpretive Statements*, p. 9. Kansas City, MO: ANA.

17. Jameton, Duties to self, p. 124.

18. American Nurses Association. 2001. *Code of Ethics for Nurses*, p. 18.

19. Ibid.

20. American Nurses Association. 1960. *Interpretation of the statements of the Code for Professional Nurses*, p. 11. New York: ANA.

21. American Nurses Association. 1926. A Suggested Code, p. 600.

22. American Nurses Association. 1985. *Code for Nurses*, p. 13.

23. Ibid., p. 19.

24. American Nurses Association. 2001. *Code of Ethics for Nurses*, Interpretive Statement 5.3, p. 19.

25. Burgess, Mary Ayers. 1928. The hospital and the nursing supply. *Transaction of the American Hospital Association*, pp. 440–41. Chicago: AHA.

26. American Nurses Association. 1985. *Code for Nurses*, p. 14.

About the Author

Marsha D.M. Fowler, PhD, MDiv, MS, RN, FAAN, is Senior Fellow and Professor of Ethics, Spirituality, and Faith Integration at Azusa Pacific University. She is a graduate of Kaiser Foundation School of Nursing (diploma), University of California at San Francisco (BS, MS), Fuller Theological Seminary (MDiv), and the University of Southern California (PhD). She has engaged in teaching and research in bioethics and spirituality since 1974. Her research interests are in the history and development of nursing ethics and the Code of Ethics for Nurses, social ethics and professions, suffering, the intersections of spirituality and ethics, and religious ethics in nursing. Dr. Fowler is also a Fellow in the American Academy of Nursing.

Provision Six

The nurse participates in establishing, maintaining, and improving healthcare environments and conditions of employment conducive to the provision of quality health care and consistent with the values of the profession through individual and collective action.

Provision Six

Linda L. Olson, PhD, RN, CNAA

An ethical work environment contributes to safe, high quality patient care as well as to patient and staff satisfaction. The 2001 ANA Code of Ethics for Nurses can aid nurses in examining the practices in their workplace, guide their actions when interacting with patients and colleagues, and assist in the assessment of the workplace ethics.

When the ANA Code was revised in 2001, a heightened emphasis on the professional responsibility for creating and maintaining an ethical work environment was incorporated, especially into the sixth provision. This provision has three sections in the form of its interpretive statements. The first section deals with the influence of the environment on moral virtues and values. The second section discusses the influence of the environment on ethical obligations. The third section discusses concepts related to nurses' interactions with colleagues, peers, and others in the workplace, as well as to their individual and collective responsibility for the healthcare environment.

Historical Context of Provision 6

Previous versions of the ANA Code of Ethics for Nurses (1968, 1976, 1985) focus on the role of the staff nurse in the hospital setting. The 2001 Code recognizes that nurses in all roles and settings face ethical issues and conflicts that should be addressed. It also recognizes the changing context within which health care is provided and nurses practice. Thus, the revised Code applies to nurses who are in practice, education, administration, research, consultation, and all other settings where nurses work, including situations of self-employment.

The Code of Ethics has historically changed in response to the social context in which nursing is practiced, and is therefore a dynamic and living document (Fowler, 1999; ANA, 2000). Both the 1976 and 1985 versions of the Code of Ethics recognized that nurses may participate in collective action as a means to achieve control of nursing practice and employment conditions that are "conducive to high quality nursing care" and to meeting the professional standards of nursing practice. Previous versions of the Code included content related to nurses' economic and general welfare. Today's healthcare environment is one in which it is imperative to attend to concerns for providing quality patient care in ways that are cost-effective. Concerns for both patient and staff safety are emphasized. In order to continue to serve as a resource for nurses in the current healthcare context, it was thought important to include a provision about the importance of the work environment as an influence on nurses' ethical and professional practice. The revised International Council of Nurses (ICN) Code of Ethics (2006) also emphasizes the role of the work environment as an influence on nurses' ethical practice. The Task Force for the revision of the Code concluded that nurses' responsibility for creating and maintaining an ethical work environment needed to receive greater attention in the 2001 version of the Code of Ethics for Nurses.

Interpretive Statement 6.1: Influence of the Environment on Moral Virtues and Values

Interpretive Statement 6.1 addresses the importance of nurse participation in constructing an environment that will contribute to the flourishing of the virtues and values central to the nursing profession and its practice. While the focus of the interpretive statement is on the influence of environment on moral virtues and values, there is an underlying interrelationship that is understood. The work environment acts upon the nurse; the nurse acts upon the work environment. The work setting can either obstruct or support nursing values and virtues. The nurse can either remain silent when the work environment is obstructive or work to change the environment. The Code is clear in its expectation of moral activism.

The interpretive statement identifies some of the values central to nursing: human dignity; well-being; and respect for persons, health, and independence. The interpretive statement also identifies some of the virtues and excellences essential to good nursing: wisdom, honesty, courage, compassion, patience, and skill. It assumes that the nurse, shaped by nursing education, brings these values, virtues, and excellences to the work setting; the nurse does not come to the work or clinical setting as a "clean slate." These values, virtues, and excellences lead some persons to choose nursing and other healthcare professions in the first place, particularly those with dispositions of helpfulness, kindness, courage, compassion, caring, and integrity. These moral virtues can be nurtured—or challenged, or thwarted—through the experiences one has in becoming a professional nurse (through the educational environment) and working in a healthcare organization.

Some ethical theories give priority to who we are morally over what we are to do. Moral character is the core of who we are as a person and is expressed in who we are and what we do, even when no one else sees. The virtues that form the basis of moral character are developed and learned throughout life from family nurturing and relationships with others. For some, these virtues are developed through faith and education, specifically the process of socialization into the values of the profession.

Although the ANA Code of Ethics does not support one specific ethical theory, virtue ethics provide some perspective on the relationship between the individual nurse's values and those of the organization and employer. The ancient Greek philosopher Aristotle described the theory of virtue ethics as habits, which are learned, providing the core of who we are as persons, in essence our moral character. In virtue ethics, moral character is learned or habituated and should not be confused with "personality traits." At the core of character is the concept of integrity. Leaders are expected to have personal and professional integrity and to exhibit behavior that is congruent with stated beliefs, or, in other words, leading by their own example, role modeling, or "walking the talk." One particularly effective way to communicate personal and professional virtue and values is through modeling them in one's behavior. When managers or colleagues recognize the contributions of a coworker by offering words of encouragement or listening to the opinions of others in a nonjudgmental way, they are demonstrating their value of respect for persons. In creating and managing an ethical work environment, organizational leaders serve to promote the personal and professional integrity of the employees by supporting a moral milieu that fosters these values and virtues.

Professional nurses make decisions that significantly affect the lives of others on a daily basis. Just as personal ethics occur within the context of relationships with others, professional ethics occurs within the context of relationships with whom one works (Gini, 2003). Although one may know the right thing to do, the context of the decision often puts nurses in ethically difficult situations. When there is a conflict between what is best for the patient versus the requirements and demands of the institution, the physician, and/or one's own self-interest, one's professional and personal integrity can be tested. Ethical behavior may require nurses to have the courage to confront their colleagues when they behaving inappropriately or in an unsafe manner. By expressing the values that underlie the profession of nursing and its practice, the Code of Ethics serves as a framework to guide nurses in their everyday practice.

Watson, in her *Ethics of Caring*, bases the Theory of Human Science and Human Care on ten carative factors. Watson refers to caring as the "essence of nursing practice," and as a "moral ideal rather than a task-oriented behavior" (Neil, 2002; p. 147). Caring is considered one of nursing's core values. As such, one must demonstrate caring in several spheres of practice, to include caring for patients, colleagues, ourselves, and the organization or employer. In Watson's *Nursing* (1999) spirituality, caring, and the nature of the interpersonal relationships nurses have with their patients are recognized as key to healing and healthy behaviors. Acting with respect, caring, and compassion applies not only to one's interactions with patients and families, but also to colleagues, co-workers, assistants, students, and others. Thus, within the context of this interpretive statement, caring is both a value and an excellence. (Within a duty-based or principle-based ethics, caring can also be considered to be a duty.)

In the context of the current healthcare environment, healthcare professionals must balance their values related to caring for patients and serving as their advocates, within the business policies of their work setting. Achieving this balance can sometimes create tension. Some work settings obstruct maintenance of nursing values, some challenge them and demand compromise. How far that compromise might go is important; compromise should ideally be integrity preserving. The tension between professional and work setting values may raise the question of whether nurses can continue to practice as morally good agents in situations where cost-constraints restrict care and staffing. Cost-cutting measures may lead to a lack of sufficient numbers of qualified and available professional nurses.

Nurses have traditionally faced situations of competing values, loyalties, and obligations within the workplace, with conflict occurring amongst these on a daily basis. In order to meet the needs of both the patient and the healthcare worker, a collaborative and supportive work environment is essential. Numerous articles have been published and studies conducted to identify the characteristics of healthy work environments. Characteristics of healthy work environments include effective leadership, interpersonal relationships and communication, as well as collaborative practice relationships among nurses and physicians (AACN, 2005). The manner in which one interacts with and relates to others, as well as the day-to-day ethical challenges and crisis-focused life and death issues, are the issues that can shape the ethical environment of the workplace. Several professional organizations and agencies, including the American Nurses Association, the Institute of Medicine, the American Association of Critical Care Nurses, and the American Organization of Nurse Executives, have identified the importance of creating a healthy and positive work environment. The American Nurses Credentialing Center (ANCC) Magnet Recognition Program gives recognition to organizations that demonstrate outstanding quality in nursing practice and provides a framework for creating cultures of excellence. The ANA Bill of Rights for Registered Nurses was developed as a policy statement with specific attention to the workplace environment (ANA, 2001).

In corroboration of the expectations of the Code of Ethics, The Bill of Rights for Registered Nurses emphasizes nurses' rights to:

- Practice in a manner that fulfills their obligations to society and to those who receive nursing care.

- Practice in environments that allow them to act in accordance with professional standards and legally authorized scopes of practice.

- A work environment that supports and facilitates ethical practice, in accordance with the Code of Ethics for Nurses and its interpretive statements.

- Freely and openly advocate for themselves and their patients, without fear of retribution.

- A work environment that is safe.

- Negotiate the conditions of employment.

In seeking out and choosing a place of employment, nurses should become familiar with the values and culture of the institution in which they seek to work. Just as individuals have their own values and principles on which to base behavior and decisions, organizations also have statements of values and a mission for which they exist. The nurse may review the organization's mission statement, organizational values, and goals when considering employment. Another way to assess the organizational culture of a company is to obtain information through talking with staff, leaders, managers, and other key players in order to obtain an impression of what type of person fits in at this organization. The way an organization's leaders treat their staff is an indicator of the organizational culture. When staff feel they are treated fairly and with respect, they translate this onto the way they treat their patients. The importance of the work environment in influencing nurses' work and patient outcomes is reflected in the concepts of organizational fit and organizational culture, mission, values, and goals. As members of a healthcare institution, nurses are expected to promote and support the organization's mission and goals. As is the case with individuals, institutions do not always live up to their stated values. It is not always possible to ascertain an institution's level of congruence with its public statements of values in advance of accepting a position.

When nurses find themselves in an environment in which they perceive a conflict between their personal and professional values and those of the institution, they first need to assess the source of that conflict. When an institution has a value structure that does not match that of the nurse, it might be better to seek employment else-where. However, when a situation arises because of an institutional failing to live up to its stated values, such as promising "high-quality patient care," but regularly suffers from nurse understaffing, that creates a conflict with the values of the pro-fession that the nurse has an obligation to attempt to correct. Where nurses works in a subpar environment and have made attempts to change it, then other avenues should be pursued depending upon the gravity of the situation.

There are several strategies that may be applied. One such strategy is to discuss the perceived conflict with the immediate supervisor and, then, to follow the appro-priate lines of communication within the employment setting. Depending on the situation, this may involve following either the nursing, medical, and/or adminis-trative chain of command in the facility. Additional strategies include reporting the situation to regulatory agencies, such as The Joint Commission or appropriate local or state health department or other agency. The Constituent Member Associations affiliated with the American Nurses Association can also provide assistance and sup-port in identifying strategies. The institution's ethics committee is also a resource for consultation and guidance when one is faced with difficult issues that adversely affect patients or staff. The most appropriate option is generally to stay in one's setting and work to change the environment, especially when patient safety and quality of care are threatened. In some cases, when changes are not forthcoming, the most appropriate strategy may be to seek employment elsewhere.

Interpretive Statement 6.2:
Influence of the Environment on Ethical Obligations

Interpretive Statement 6.2 recognizes that the policies and practices of a work environment have an influence on ethical obligations. The professional atmosphere of an organization influences employee behavior and beliefs, and, thus, ethical decision making. The organizational culture is reflected in way things are done in the work setting. It consists of the norms and values, as well as the mechanisms by which the organization carries out its work. Policies, procedures, conditions of employment, structures for decision making, and the types of behaviors that are supported constitute the culture of an organization. The climate of an organization is judged by employee perceptions of how the policies and procedures are actu-ally carried out, along with their effectiveness. It influences how one feels to be a member of that particular organization. One crucial aspect of an organization is its ethical climate, a concept that can be defined as how employees perceive the behaviors and practices associated with how ethical issues are handled (Olson 1995). Brown (1990) described five conditions that must be present in the work environment in order for awareness, reflection, and discussion about ethical issues to occur. These conditions are (a) power (the right to having the information needed to understand a situation, as well as to say what needs to be said), (b) trust (the confidence to disagree with others, without fear of reprisal), (c) inclusion (those with an interest in the decision are included in the process), (d) role flexibility (the ability to take different points of view, and to change it based on additional information), and (e) inquiry (an atmosphere of questioning and learning).

Interpretive Statement 6.3: Responsibility for the Healthcare Environment

Interpretive Statement 6.3 addresses nurses' individual and collective responsibility for contributing to the healthcare environment. Each individual nurse has a role in creating an ethical environment. Nurses, as both members of society and healthcare professionals, face ethical issues and dilemmas on a daily basis. These range from basic issues, such as treating colleagues, patients, and families with respect and truth-telling, and patient advocacy, to more complex issues, such as those associated with end-of-life care. Inherent within these issues are competing loyalties among the best interests of patients and the obligations toward physicians and the employing organization. Provision 2 makes clear the imperative that the first obligation is to the patient (see Chapter 2). In reality, this is often difficult, particularly when one is faced with balancing multiple obligations in the workplace.

Each individual nurse has a role in creating and contributing to an ethical environment. It is recommended that nurses assess their own values as well as those of the organization in order to determine whether they will be supported in their roles as patient advocates and moral agents (Hamric, 1999; Maier-Lorentz, 2000). What does an ethical work environment mean, and what are its characteristics? In light of the current worldwide shortage of nurses, as well as individual staffing shortages in many institutions, the importance of nurses maintaining an ethical work environment is unsurpassed.

There are primarily two strategies for solving the current shortage of qualified and available nursing personnel. One strategy is to increase the supply of professional nurses through enhancing the capacity of nursing schools to accept more students. This supply-side strategy also requires an increase in the numbers of qualified faculty. The second strategy, a demand-side strategy, is to improve the workplace environment, thereby retaining nurses in the organization, as well as in the profession. Changing the culture of the workplace environment to one that demonstrates increased recognition and rewards for nurses who excel in practice will ultimately improve the quality of patient outcomes and enhance nurse recruitment and retention.

One way to promote an ethical environment is to use the ANA Code of Ethics for Nurses as a resource for guidance. In order to use the Code as an organizational resource, it should be readily available to all nurses. Awareness of the Code and how to use it to guide practice is increased through reviewing it during facility orientations and educational programs, incorporating it into job descriptions, and including it as a component of the philosophy and conceptual framework for the practice of nursing within the organization. When nurses are encouraged to think about how their practice reflects the Code, they are more likely to develop a sense of ethical awareness and view it as a source of support when faced with ethical issues and conflicts. To engage in ethical decisions, nurses must be knowledgeable about the issues involved and how the decision-making process works, as well as how to use organizational mechanisms, such as hospital ethics committees, consultation resources, and formal and informal lines of communication. It is also important that nurses have input into organizational decision making and have the opportunity to participate with policy and procedure committees.

The demands of the Code that nurses actively participate in establishing and maintaining the moral environment have been reinforced by recent research on the necessity of "speaking up." The Silence Kills study identified seven categories of "crucial conversations" that, when avoided, can profoundly affect patient care. These categories are: broken rules, mistakes, lack of support, incompetence, poor teamwork, disrespect, and micromanagement (Maxfield et al, 2005). Indeed, speaking up is a moral obligation. This research evidence supports the moral importance of expressing concern regarding untoward behavior, decisions, or actions on the part of colleagues and the consequences for patient care of not doing so.

Role of the Manager in Creating an Ethical Environment

Perhaps the most important role in creating, enhancing, and maintaining an ethical environment is that of the first-line manager. The nurse manager is not only responsible for safe patient care that is cost-effective and of high quality, and also for assuring that the nurses who deliver that care are competent and adhere to professional standards of practice. The nurse manager plays a key role in retaining qualified nurses, as well as in promoting their job satisfaction. There is already literature that provides evidence of a relationship between levels of nurse staffing and patient outcomes (Aiken et al., 2002). Research has also shown that employees who perceive their leaders as basing their decisions on ethical values and practices are more satisfied with their jobs (Vitell and Davis, 1990). Nurse managers, who are in first-line positions in hospital or other healthcare settings, are perceived as having the most crucial and difficult positions by virtue of being the liaisons between the direct caregivers and the administration. Conflicts often arise between the nurse managers' obligations to their staff, their patients, and their employers. When such conflicts arise, it is important that mechanisms are in place to facilitate open communication and support in an atmosphere where issues can be addressed and resolved appropriately. The goals of safe, high-quality care and satisfied patients, employees, and physicians, are considered to be important organizational outcomes. Balanced reports and scorecards to accrediting agencies, employer groups, and the public highlight these aspects of a healthcare organization's mission and goals.

Promoting a nonthreatening atmosphere in which nurses and others can mutually express and share their concerns is an important component of an ethical work environment. In addition, such communication helps employees perceive they have a role in the success and viability of the organization as well. Provision 6 also addresses the role of accountability. Just as individual professional nurses are expected to be accountable for their practice, managers must clearly communicate the responsibilities expected of their staff and hold them accountable for their performance.

Case Example 1

Collaborative Practice Relationships

A large academic medical center established a mechanism whereby nurses and physicians met regularly to discuss and plan the treatment goals and interventions for their patients. In this atmosphere of mutual problem-solving, communication, respect for each others' viewpoints, and sharing of observations and assessments, nurses felt they were an equal part of the patient care team. As a result of this collaborative mechanism of shared decision making, nurses also reported fewer instances of moral distress and outrage. Moral outrage is an emotional response associated with the inability to do what one perceives as the right thing to do as a result of organizational constraints. A collaborative and supportive environment is essential in order to effectively meet the needs of patients, families, and the community.

Three months ago a new, extremely well-known specialist physician was hired and brought a physician assistant with him. The medical staff is elated that this physician has agreed to join them and see him as both a clinical plus and public relations boost for the hospital. From the start, the physician made rounds with his physician assistant and asked that the nurses not participate because the physician "did not want to be delayed in his rounds" by the presence of nurses. Free communication exists between the physician and the physician's assistant, but not with the nurses. The nurses have been instructed that if they wish to communicate with the physician they must go through the physician assistant. The nurses have become increasingly frustrated and feel cut out of patient care. They believe that the level of medical care remains high, but they also perceive that the goal of high-quality nursing care is being obstructed. Furthermore, they resent having to communicate with a physician assistant instead of the physician, and have proceeded to contact the physician directly. This has angered the physician and hardened the position he is taking. The nurse manager and the unit CNS have both spoken with the physician, but he will not budge. The second time they attempt to raise concerns on behalf of the nursing staff, the physician becomes imperious and demeaning. What, if anything, should be done, individually or collectively, by the nurses to remedy this situation? ■

Case Example 2
Compassionate and Respectful Interactions with Students, Mentoring, Role Modeling, and Modeling of the Profession's Core Values

A nursing school initiates a mentoring program whereby all undergraduate students meet in assigned groups with a faculty mentor each semester in their program. This mechanism is a way to provide students (and future nurses) with a sense of empowerment and a source of support, as well as permitting them to express themselves in a safe environment, without fear of reprisal. It is also a means by which the values of the profession can be transmitted. This mechanism provides students with a forum of trust and respect for expressing their feelings and of preserving their dignity. However, one group of junior students is experiencing distress. Their mentor, a senior faculty member and department chairperson, has an outside business and asks for "volunteers" to work in his "community health center," predominantly funded by federal grants, where, they are expected to do unsupervised well-child health assessments. The students believe that refusing to volunteer will have negative consequences, so they comply. The students feel inadequate to the task, but the faculty person states that this is "related clinical experience that is supervised." In addition, one of the students found the grant proposal on the internet and discovered that it contains provisions in the budget for registered nurses to conduct these assessments. This is a powerful faculty member; other faculty refuse to discuss this with the students. What ought the students do? ■

Conditions of Employment

A component of Provision 6 is that conditions of employment must be conducive to the provision of quality patient care and consistent with the professional values related to individual and collective action. As employees, nurses have a right to have input into decisions related to conditions of employment, professional practice, and patient care. This not only contributes to nurse job satisfaction, but also to organizational commitment and retention. When nurses perceive the conditions in their practice setting as unfavorable, inequitable, and unsafe, they may seek representation through collective action, including collective bargaining as a way to assure their opinions about workplace conditions and patient care are heard. The most important consideration here is the relationship that nurses as direct caregivers have with management and administration.

The use of the term "collective action" encompasses a variety of mechanisms by which nurses participate in organizational decisions regarding their workplace conditions. The formal mechanisms associated with collective bargaining, workplace advocacy programs, and shared governance provide ways to empower nurses to participate in decisions affecting their work conditions and patient care (Green and Jordan, 2004; Williams, 2004; Budd et al, 2004).

A collective bargaining agreement is a negotiated legal mechanism that results in empowering nurses so that they have a voice in decisions that affect their work conditions and control over their practice. When conditions within the employment setting are perceived as unacceptable and nurses and administrators do not trust or respect each other in ways that facilitate effective communication and problem-solving, nurses sometimes turn to unionization as a means of gaining negotiating power. Nurses seek representation by unions for many reasons, including solving problems regarding wages, workload and staffing, and addressing issues related to practice, such as safe, quality patient care and an ethical environment in which to work. Admittedly, collective bargaining has sometimes focused on benefits to nurses and staff, to the exclusion of concerns for the ethical environment. The reasons for collective action, in whatever form it takes, fall into two main categories: workplace issues that affect the nurse alone (e.g., wages, benefits, hours, treatment) and those that affect nursing care and patient welfare (e.g., staffing patterns, participation in decision making, governance). The collective bargaining contract becomes a tool whereby nurses can achieve positive conditions in the workplace through a negotiated process. It is incumbent upon nurses to press the collective bargaining unit to attend to the ethical environment of the workplace, in addition to other concerns. Negotiating a collective bargaining contract may result in improved conditions of employment for nurses and provide a means to achieve goals that result in improved patient care outcomes as well. These goals are of interest also to nurse managers and the organization. Whereas the values inherent within the Code include caring, respect, trust, and collaboration, the process of collective bargaining guarantees a legal contract between the two parties that can support these values.

In order to ensure that the contract negotiations stay within an ethical framework, it helps to view the process as one in which nurses are achieving the best possible conditions of employment for themselves, while also creating policies and standards that result in improved patient care. For example, when nurses negotiate to set staffing standards as a component of their collective bargaining contract, they are also creating an environment that provides safe, high-quality patient care and supports nurse recruitment and retention.

The term "workplace advocacy" refers to programs aimed at facilitating nurses' involvement in workplace decisions that affect patient care and providing individual nurses with resources to help them to be advocates for themselves in their work environments. These strategies may be part of a program that involves professional organizations at the local, state, and national levels. The Center for American Nurses (CAN) is a formal program of the American Nurses Association. It provides various services to assist nurses in self-advocacy through focusing on staffing, workflow design, the physical environment, and personal, social, and organizational factors.

Shared governance is another formal structure that achieves the goal of sharing decision making through mechanisms such as nurse practice councils in which nurses from all levels of the organization contribute to decisions concerning the work environment. Other shared governance councils may focus on policies, procedures, research, quality improvement, education, recruitment, and retention.

In the ideal world, nurses and their managers and administrators would always collaborate successfully on issues related to workplace conditions and patient care policies in order to achieve mutually satisfactory outcomes. Shared governance models embody the concept of participatory decision making. Mechanisms of shared governance include staff bylaws and structures, such as councils, that involve employees in developing policies and procedures, build collaborative relationships among staff and management, and foster organizational autonomy. Shared governance is viewed as a strategy that provides mechanisms for empowering nurses. It is also considered a key indicator of excellence, as embodied by the achievements of Magnet hospitals. Shared governance models and collective bargaining agreements can co-exist in the same organization, so long as union leaders work along with managers and staff nurses to create the model (Budd et al, 2004; O'Grady, 2001). This is one type of systems-level organizational culture change that can improve the environment in which nurses provide patient care (Institute of Medicine, 2004).

Shared Governance and Collective Bargaining in the Same Hospital

The use of shared governance and collective bargaining in the same institution can be fruitful. For example, the nurses at one large academic medical center hospital originally organized using collective bargaining for purposes of improving their wages and benefits. After that, the nurses stated their desire to have input into decisions on patient care issues and other polices and procedures that affected practice. They also wanted to be recognized for their expertise and competence, as well as for their seniority in the hospital. As a result of collaboration among managers and staff, as well as the desire of the hospital to pursue Magnet Recognition status, a decision was made to establish unit-based councils as a mechanism for staff nurses to have input into decisions about patient care. With the belief that empowering nurses in decision making would also result in improved patient outcomes, the leaders of the collective bargaining unit, the nurse leaders and the administrators met to discuss concepts of shared governance.

Although direct care nurses were already involved in several committees throughout the hospital, these discussions resulted in the creation of a professional practice model that included unit-based councils, with representatives who were members of councils concerned with quality council, nurse practice, education and professional development, research, and recruitment and retention. A staff nurse served as chairs of each council and participated in the overall nursing leadership council, which also included nursing administrators. Though development of this council, surveys indicated that nurses felt empowered to make changes in their work environment that ultimately resulted in improved patient and nurse satisfaction. Notice the rich variety of mechanisms and structures that were put in place in this situation. With these changes, nurses reported feeling they had control over their practice and autonomy in their decision making. Through the collaborative relationship that had developed among clinical nurses and management, a level of mutual respect and trust was present. Clinical nurses perceived they had real input and participation in decisions related to their roles in patient care. When it was time for their application and site visit, they were successful in achieving Magnet recognition. This success was attributed to the collective bargaining commitment of nurses and the nursing administrative leadership to work collaboratively toward building a shared governance structure. Although conflicts still occurred, there was a mechanism in place for voicing of concerns and providing input in an atmosphere of respect and renewed trust.

The American Nurses Association, through its various programs and structures, advocates for safe working conditions for both nurses and patients through collective bargaining, workplace advocacy (both formal and informal), and in serving as a resource providing guidance for nurses with practice-related problems. Through its formal position statements, Code of Ethics, Bill of Rights, Scope and Standards of Practice (ANA, 2004), Social Policy Statement (ANA, 2003), and legislative action, this professional nurses association serves as an advocate for nurses and patients. In addition, the Magnet Recognition Program developed and administered by the American Nurses Credentialing Center serves to recognize healthcare organizations that demonstrate excellence in nursing care and practice (ANCC, 2007). The Magnet Recognition Program serves as a klieg light sweeping the dark skies of Hollywood saying "Look at us; this is where you want to be." In summary, Provision 6 is about the role of the nurse in creating, promoting, and maintaining an ethical environment for practice. The three interpretive statements that explicate this provision address the influence of the work environment on nurses' ethical practice, as well as the role of the nurse in contributing to the creation of an ethical environment for practice.

References

All online references were accessed in December 2007.

Aiken, L.H., S.P. Clarke, D.M. Sloane, J. Sochalski, and J.H. Silber, 2002. Hospital nurse staffing and patient mortality, nurse burnout, and job dissatisfaction. *Journal of the American Medical Association* 288(16): 1987–93.

American Association of Critical-Care Nurses. 2005. AACN Standards for establishing and sustaining healthy work environments. www.aacn.org.

American Nurses Association. 2000. Code of Ethics Project Task Force. A New Code of Ethics for Nurses. *American Journal of Nursing* 100(7): 69–72.

American Nurses Association. 2001. *Bill of Rights for Registered Nurses.* Washington, DC: American Nurses Publishing.

American Nurses Association. 2001. *Code of Ethics for Nurses with Interpretive Statements.* Washington, DC: American Nurses Publishing.

American Nurses Association. 2003. *Nursing's Social Policy Statement.* Washington, DC: American Nurses Publishing.

American Nurses Association. 2004. *Nursing: Scope and Standards of Practice.* Washington, DC: Nursesbooks.org.

American Nurses Credentialing Center. 2007. Magnet Recognition Program: Recognizing excellence in nursing service. http://www.nursecredentialing.org/magnet/index.html.

Arwedson, I.L., S. Roos, and A. Björklund. 2007. Constituents of healthy workplaces. *Work* 28(1): 3–11.

Brown, M.T. 1990. *Working Ethics.* San Francisco: Jossey-Bass.

Budd, K.W., L.S. Warino, and M.E. Patton. 2004. Traditional and non-traditional collective bargaining: Strategies to improve the patient care environment. *Online Journal of Issues in Nursing,* 31 January, 9(1).

Fowler, M.D. 1999. Relic or resource? The Code for Nurses. *American Journal of Nursing* 99(3): 56–57.

Gates, D. 2006. Changing the work environment to promote wellness: A focus group study. *AAOHN Journal* 54(12): 515–20.

Gini, A. 2003. *My Job, My Self.* NY: Routledge.

Green, A., and C. Jordan. 2004. Common denominators: Shared governance and work place advocacy-strategies for nurses to gain control over their practice. *Online Journal of Issues in Nursing,* 31 January, 9(1).

Hamric, A.B. 1999. The nurse as a moral agent in modern health care. *Nursing Outlook* 47(3): 106.

Institute of Medicine. 2004. *Keeping Patients Safe: Transforming the Work Environment of Nurses.* Washington, DC: National Academies Press.

International Council of Nurses (ICN) 2000. *ICN Code of Ethics for Nurses.* Geneva, Switzerland: ICN.

Kane-Urrabazo C. 2006. Management's role in shaping organizational culture. *Journal of Nursing Management* 14(3; Apr): 188–94.

Maier-Lorentz, M.M. 2000. Creating your own ethical environment. *Nursing Forum* 35(3), 25–28.

Maxfield, D.J. Grenny, R. McMillan, K. Patterson, and A. Switzler. 2005. *Silence Kills: The Seven Crucial Conversations for Healthcare.* http://www.aacn.org/ aacn/pubpolcy.nsf/Files/ SilenceKillsExecSum/$file/SilenceKillsExecSum.pdf.

Neil, R.M. 2002. Jean Watson: Philosophy and science of caring. In *Nursing Theorists and their Work.* 5th ed., pp. 145–64. Springfield, MO: Mosby.

Oandasan, I. 2007. Teamwork and healthy workplaces: Strengthening the links for deliberation and action through research and policy. *Healthcare Papers* 7, Special Issue: 98–103.

O'Grady, T.P. 2001. Collective bargaining: The union as partner. *Nursing Management* 32(6), 30–32.

Olson, L.L. 1995. Hospital nurses' perceptions of the ethical climate of their work setting. *Image: The Journal of Nursing Scholarship* 30(4): 345–49.

Patterson, K., J. Grenny, A. Switzler, and R. McMillan. 2002. *Crucial Conversations: Tools for Talking When Stakes Are High.* New York: McGraw-Hill.

Reina, M.L., and C. Barden. 2007. Creating a healthy workplace. Trust: the foundation for team collaboration and healthy work environments. *AACN Advanced Critical Care* 18(2; Apr–Jun): 103–8.

Ulrich, B.T., R. Lavandero, K.A. Hart, D. Woods, J. Legget, and D. Taylor. 2006. Critical care nurses' work environments: A baseline status report. *Critical Care Nurse* 26(5), 46–57.

Vitell, S.J., and D.L. Davis. 1990. The relationship between ethics and job satisfaction: An empirical investigation. *Journal of Business Ethics* 9, 489–94.

Watson, J. 1988. *Nursing: Human Science and Human Care: A Theory of Nursing.* New York: National League for Nursing.

Watson, J., and M.A. Ray. 1989. *The Ethics of Care and the Ethics of Cure: Synthesis in Chronicity.* New York: National League for Nursing.

Williams, K.O. 2004. Ethics and collective bargaining: Calls to action. *Online Journal of Issues in Nursing* 23 July.

About the Author

Linda L. Olson, PhD, RN, CNAA, is currently Professor and Dean of the School of Nursing at North Park University in Chicago, Illinois. Previously, she taught courses in healthcare policy and economics, leadership, and nursing service administration at the graduate and undergraduate levels as an Associate Professor at St. Xavier University in Chicago. She has prior experience in nursing service administration, practice, and consultation. Dr. Olson received her PhD and MBA from the University of Illinois at Chicago, and her baccalaureate and master's degrees in nursing from Northern Illinois University. Her area of research interest is the work environment, particularly focusing on organizational culture and ethics. As part of her dissertation work, she developed the research instrument, the Hospital Ethical Climate Survey, which has also been used by several researchers, nurses, and others in the United States and internationally. She was a member of the ANA Task Force to Revise the Code of Ethics, as well as the Congress on Nursing Practice and Economics, and has held numerous leadership positions at local, state, and national levels. In addition, she serves as an appraiser for the Magnet Recognition Program.

Guide to the Code of Ethics for Nurses

Provision
Seven

The nurse participates in the advancement of the
profession through contributions to practice, education,
administration, and knowledge development.

Provision Seven

Theresa S. Drought, PhD, RN, and
Elizabeth G. Epstein, PhD, RN

Provision History

Nursing has changed tremendously in the last twenty years. Advanced degrees at the master's and doctoral levels, as well as advanced practice nursing, have created expanding opportunities for nurses to contribute to health care, education, research, public awareness, and health and social policy in unprecedented ways. Nursing research has blossomed. Nurses hold prominent positions, both appointed and elected, in government, philanthropy, and social policy institutes. One of these, the National Institutes of Health's National Institute for Nursing Research (NINR), is focused on nursing research. Nursing issues are prominent on the agendas of Congress, the United Nations, and such influential private organizations as the Robert Wood Johnson Foundation, the Pew Charitable Trusts, and the RAND Corporation.

In the initial review of the Code of Ethics of 1985, it was recognized that the previous Provision 7 ("The nurse participates in activities that contribute to the ongoing development of the professional's body of knowledge.") required expansion and clarification for several reasons. First, this provision placed emphasis on the importance of knowledge development without acknowledging the many other ways nurses can advance the nursing profession. The current formulation recognizes the multifaceted complexity of contemporary nursing practice and seeks to make the provision relevant to nurses in all settings and roles. Second, the individual nurse has just as much of an obligation to the profession as the profession has to the individual nurse. This reciprocity was not addressed in the previous formulation, but it is a significant aspect of the current formulation. Third, education, practice, and administration, as well as knowledge development are inherently interdependent. Little forward movement in the profession can be made if new knowledge is not translated into practice. Educators must be aware of the realities of practice as well as the latest advances in research. Administrators must create an environment that is supportive of the ongoing educational needs of nurses and conducive to rapid implementation of innovation. Quality patient care is dependent upon the development of effective educational methods; efficient, cost-effective system administration, and research to guide the provision of nursing care. Finally, patient well-being is dependent upon a vibrant, evolving nursing profession that is responsive and able to anticipate the emerging needs of society and healthcare systems. The profession can only advance through the participation of nurses who are open to learning, and incorporating new knowledge. Clearly, the future of the profession is dependent upon more than the work of a few individuals; it requires the active engagement of all nurses.

Provision Content

Provision 7 challenges the nurse to participate in the profession's contributions to society by being actively engaged with its progress and development. One purpose of the Code is to reinforce the bonds between the individual who chooses to enter the nursing profession, the practice of the individual nurse, and the social roles and obligations of nurses within society. This provision creates a moral link between the nurse as a person, the individual practice of the nurse, and the nursing profession as a whole. This link is necessary in order for the nurse to hold a coherent sense of professional obligation that complements the individual's sense of self.

Note how Provisions 4, 5, 8, and 9 are closely linked in Provision 7. The nurse as a moral agent is described in Provision 5. Provision 4 describes the moral obligations of the nurse as a practitioner. Provision 8 describes the nurse's moral obligation to society. Provision 9 describes the responsibilities of the nursing profession to both the individual nurse and society in general. Provision 7 provides the necessary linkage between individual competence and evolving professional standards of practice, in addition to giving nurses a responsive and collaborative role in health policy for the overall advancement of the profession. It also clarifies the interdependent relationship between the ability of the nursing profession to contribute to society and the well-being and development of the individual nurse and the profession as a whole. Just as a nurse who is undertrained, unsupported, and isolated cannot contribute to the patient's well-being, a profession that is undeveloped, fragmented, and lacking in the commitment and support of its practitioners will be limited in its ability to benefit society.

It is not expected that the individual nurse will be proficient in all areas of nursing or engaged with each facet of development required for advancement of the profession (education, practice, administration, and knowledge development). However, the nurse cannot afford to be indifferent to the advancement of the profession; our systems of health care change rapidly and nursing as a profession must anticipate and adapt to these changes in order to meet the needs of patients. The expectation laid out in Provision 7 is that the individual nurses will bring their talents and experience to the ongoing conversation about nursing practice and standards that is needed to advance the profession as a whole. Individual competence cannot be maintained without the nurse's awareness of changes in professional practice, standards, and health policy. Advancements in these areas cannot be attained without input from all areas of nursing practice. The demands of nursing exceed the capacity of any individual working in isolation. The interdependence between nurses, their practice, the profession, and the many facets of nursing knowledge is implicit in both Provisions 7 and 9.

Interpretive Statements

The three interpretive statements are like the layers of an onion and serve to amplify the meaning of Provision 7 and illustrate its application to nursing practice. Each exposes a different layer of involvement for the nurse. It is this layered component of practice that provides for a vibrant, flourishing profession. As you peel back the layers, you expose the center of nursing—patient care. Yet without these outer layers to protect it, the center could not survive. So, while the initial provisions of the Code explicitly focus on patient care as the center of nursing, succeeding provisions also have the patient at the center.

The first interpretive statement directs the nurse to the outermost layer of interaction between the profession and society; it calls on the nurse to be actively involved in health policy and the organizations that serve as an interface between nursing practice and the public. The second interpretive statement directs the nurse to the regulation and scope of individual professional practice; it calls on the nurse to be actively involved in the development and implementation of professional standards. The third interpretive statement shields the center of nursing; it directs the nurse to develop, adapt, and utilize the research necessary for the provision of safe and effective patient care.

Interpretive Statement 7.1: Advancing the Profession through Active Involvement in Nursing and in Healthcare Policy

There are many ways to be involved in nursing and healthcare policy inside and outside the work environment. A minimal approach in the work environment would be to incorporate activities related to standards, quality initiatives, and the results of nursing research into direct patient care. Programs such as The National Patient Safety Goals and the National Database of Nursing Quality Indicators provide standards and tools to guide practice as well as encourage improvements in patient safety and quality care. At a higher level, nurses can conduct research to collect outcome data for establishing better standards and practices. Institutional participation in programs such as Magnet Recognition or the AACN Synergy Model serve to both utilize and inform health policy and patient care standards. Research conducted by nurses provides the necessary linkage between nursing education, staffing, and patient safety and outcomes (Aiken et al, 2003; Rogers et al, 2004, Rothschild et al, 2006).

Some nurses may feel they wouldn't know where to begin in engaging with public policy. However, utilizing the knowledge of health issues gained from nursing when carrying out civic responsibilities, engaging friends and family in informed discussions on health policy matters, exercising the right to vote, informing oneself about legislative and ballot issues, and writing to elected representatives on issues related to nursing can have a significant effect on health policy. At a slightly higher level of involvement, there are several avenues open to the nurse, such as providing expert testimony at legislative hearings, participating in the political action committees of professional associations, coordinating community health programs or education campaigns related to issues affecting nursing. Non-healthcare forums also benefit from nursing involvement; nurses make important contributions through participation on local school boards and regional or national advocacy groups addressing environmental and economic issues affecting society generally. Finally, nurses must strive to become active participants at the highest levels of healthcare policy in this country by running for elected office, taking leadership positions at health policy agencies, and researching and writing about issues affecting health policy.

These types of activities bring the nursing perspective to the forefront and help to advance the profession in at least two ways. First, it makes nurses' contributions to health care and patients both tangible and visible which helps to promote the value of nursing in the eyes of the public and other healthcare professionals. Second, recognition of nurses as valuable, contributing participants in health policy increases public support of the profession which will serve to strengthen nursing's effectiveness.

Interpretive Statement 7.2: Advancing the Profession by Developing, Maintaining, and Implementing Professional Standards in Clinical, Administrative, and Educational Practice

A hallmark of professionalism is self-management and -regulation; commitment to these activities is necessary for a vital, flourishing nursing practice. Allowing others to mandate the requirements or establish the boundaries of professional practice does not serve nurses or the patients who benefit from nursing care. Nurses must be the primary architects of the standards that define professional practice.

Again, there are multiple ways to meet the obligation to advance the profession as detailed in this interpretive statement. At a minimum, knowing and adhering to the professional standards applicable to the nurse's practice setting and role meets this obligation. The advancement of the profession can be attained by the conscientious practice, innovation, and refinement of each individual in accord with established standards and guidelines. Peer review creates accountability mechanisms linking individual practice to professional standards. Self-regulation is a hallmark of professionalism and key to advancement. Self-regulation includes holding one's self and peers accountable for meeting the standards of the profession. A mid-level commitment could be met by the nurse's involvement with the development of standards within a particular practice setting; participation in workplace quality committees and shared governance systems; or the collection and utilization of nurse sensitive patient care data. A slightly higher level of commitment could be met by providing commentary on legislative (the Nurse Practice Acts), regulatory (Medicare, Medicaid, JCAHO), or organizational (ANA and other professional organizations) proposals to change standards or introduce guidelines affecting nursing practice. Finally, nurses can meet this obligation by (a) educating other nurses to utilize practice standards and hold them accountable for doing so, (b) conducting research on the efficacy of nursing interventions, and (c) engaging in healthcare system evaluation and design and implementing healthcare systems of care that are based on sound standards of practice.

Guide to the Code of Ethics for Nurses

Interpretive Statement 7.3: Advancing the Profession through Knowledge Development, Dissemination, and Application to Practice

Nursing combines the art of caring with the science of health care. The nursing process is dependent upon theoretically sound and scientifically proven methods that embrace the goals of nursing: the prevention of illness, the alleviation of suffering, and the protection, promotion, and restoration of health in the care of individuals, families, groups, and communities. Research on the efficacy of existing programs and new ways of understanding disease, health, the human response to illness, and innovations in nursing care are necessary.

At first blush, it could be construed that this provision is quite demanding and requires nurses to be actively engaged in research. In truth, maintaining a competent practice combined with ongoing self-education and the utilization of results from nursing research assures that this requirement is realized. In the most basic sense, this provision can be met by conscientiously reading nursing journals to be aware of new approaches in health care, incorporating research-based interventions into professional duties, replacing outdated practices with new ones that have proven efficacy, attending clinical conferences, and remaining open to change in the work setting. At a higher level of involvement, the nurse could participate in journal clubs, practice development committees, or regional specialty organizations to learn about new findings; facilitate nursing research in the work setting; or review current literature when developing policies, procedures, and programs. Finally, the nurse can actively engage in knowledge development by conducting formal, independent, or collaborative research to find solutions to problems encountered at work and contributing to the literature that supports nursing practice.

Applying Provision 7

The following examples demonstrate how, in a wide variety of everyday nursing practices, this provision might be applied.

Case Example 1

Utilizing Particular Expertise

Elaine has been a clinical staff nurse in a busy neurology unit for the past six years. She is dedicated to her work and has developed especially good skills in working with families to communicate with and care for their loved ones who are patients in the unit. She has pursued educational opportunities to continue to develop this expertise and is active in the regional chapter of a neurology specialty organization.

There are several ways that Elaine could advance the nursing profession through leadership as discussed in Interpretive Statement 7.1. She could serve as a mentor for new nurses in the neurology unit who are learning how to teach family members to provide care for their loved ones. She could coordinate a collaborative effort with other nurses, social workers, and physicians (see Provision 8) to create an educational in-service on techniques effective in teaching families how to provide daily care. She could work within the hospital system to amend the discharge documentation, so that it includes specific competencies families must be taught prior to a patient's discharge.

Elaine could also extend her leadership into the health policy arena. She could provide testimony at legislative and budgetary hearings regarding state and federal support programs for the neurologically impaired. Her knowledge and unique perspective on the needs of family members providing care to neurologically injured patients would be a valuable contribution to decisions on programs affecting this population. In these ways, Elaine would be taking the lead in improving care for neurology patients and advancing the profession by exemplifying nursing's unique abilities in caring for this population.

Elaine's activities provide challenges and opportunities for other nurses as well. Elaine's manager is affected by what Elaine does on the unit and in the public arena. Interpretive Statements 7.1 and 7.2 acknowledge that nursing administrators should "foster an employment environment that facilitates nurses' ethical integrity and professionalism" as well as "establish, maintain, and promote conditions of employment that enables nurses...to practice in accord with accepted standards of nursing practice." In this way, Elaine's manager is pivotal to the utilization of knowledge on the unit. In an effort to make the most of Elaine's interests and skills, the nurse manager of the unit could involve Elaine in writing a hospital policy addressing educational programs with families. The profession is advanced when efforts to promote unit standards of nursing care are formalized in these types of guidelines. Involving other nurses in these processes can create a unit culture that values both individual expertise and shared development of practice.

The commitment on the part of a manager who engages staff in these activities creates a culture of excellence that can influence administrative decisions in the unit and the larger organization. The nurse manager recognizes the fact that teaching families how to feed, dress, and move the patient takes time and practice, but she prioritizes this teaching as an important aspect of nursing care. The profession is advanced when staffing decisions accommodate the time needed for this type of teaching to be accomplished. The manager's decisions have the potential to influence broader organizational policies as the values of nursing expertise and effective practice are recognized and supported.

The organization can also be directly or indirectly involved in Elaine's activities outside of the unit. If Elaine chooses to become involved in the health policy arena, she may need some flexibility in her work schedule. This can present a dilemma for the manager who is charged with seeing to the needs of the patients on the unit. However, the administration's support of Elaine's activities has the potential to benefit patients indirectly, advance the nursing profession generally, and provide positive public relations for the organization. Accommodating her schedule and publicizing her activities advances the culture of professionalism within the organization by explicitly acknowledging the contributions of nursing. ■

Case Example 2

The Nursing Instructor and the Struggling Student

Melissa is an instructor in the Nursing Skills Lab. She notices that a fourth-year student has fallen behind in her assignments and is not demonstrating competence in her clinical nursing skills. As outlined in Interpretive Statement 7.1, nurse educators "have a specific responsibility to enhance students' commitment to professional and civic values." The way Melissa chooses to interact with this and other students should be guided by Provision 7. Interacting with her students in a respectful and professional manner will influence their perception of professional behavior and can serve to advance or hold back the profession. A professionally responsible way for Melissa to address the student's difficulties would be to contact her outside of the lab in order to discuss why she has fallen behind and what needs to be done to correct the problem. By doing this, the student is acknowledged as a valued member of the class while being held accountable for her work. Melissa demonstrates her commitment to professional values through the sensitivity and professionalism with which she approaches her students as well as the way she holds them accountable. The student and Melissa both have important obligations that affect the advancement of the profession; the student's commitment to the nursing profession may be strengthened by knowing that Melissa is an advocate who will help her work through problems. Modeling ways of problem solving, providing supportive and respectful help, and maintaining boundaries of accountability, demonstrate a skill-set the student may draw upon in the future.

However, Interpretive Statement 7.2 also states that the nurse educator should promote and maintain standards of nursing education and should ensure that nursing graduates are fully prepared and competent. Keeping this in mind, Melissa has some serious responsibilities to consider. As stated in Provision 2, Melissa's primary responsibility is to the patient, so this commitment affects how she handles students' difficulties in skills lab. There are several courses of action that could be followed: she could coach the student, give her extra time to complete assignments when necessary, or work with her on a remedial basis; she could fail the student for this course and allow her to repeat it; or she could recommend that the student be released from the program. Melissa's actions will depend in large part on the level of the student's commitment and ability. What is most important, however, is that, whichever option is followed, the standards and professionalism of nursing practice are upheld. ■

Case Example 3

Complacency in the NICU

Deborah is a newborn intensive care (NICU) nurse. She is skilled at feeding and caring for medically stable infants, but is much less proficient with infants who are critically ill or whose condition changes rapidly. Deborah has a reputation in the NICU that she can teach almost any infant to take oral feedings. As one physician says, "She can successfully feed a rock." She almost never reads the professional journals and argues that her hands-on experience is more relevant than any research article could ever be. Several of her colleagues agree. They say, "What's the use, anyway? There are no incentives to read articles and use what we learn on this unit!"

The manager in the NICU is distressed to overhear this conversation, especially since a recent analysis showed that this NICU's mortality rates are moderately worse than other units of similar size and acuity. She resubmits a request to hire a Clinical Nurse Specialist (CNS) that she had submitted six months earlier and drafts a report to the nursing vice president to support her request citing the urgency of the situation. ■

Guide to the Code of Ethics for Nurses

There are several questions to ask:

- Do the attitudes of Deborah and the other nurses in the unit advance the profession?

- What are the obligations of the manager and the future CNS in this situation?

- Could the unit mortality rate be decreased if the nurses took a more active role in advancing the profession?

Although she provides excellent care for some infants and may even be revered for her ability to feed the difficult ones, Deborah is not upholding Provision 7. While it is not necessary for Deborah and her colleagues to participate actively in knowledge development if they lack the preparation, skill, or inclination, they are responsible for disseminating and applying new knowledge in their practice. Despite the fact that Deborah has not found research to be relevant, she still has valuable input to share, so long as she has read and seriously critiqued the articles. When reading a research article, it is important for the nurse to critique the methods and results because the utility and practicality of the findings must be evaluated. It is also important, however, to think more deeply about the implications of the findings. Is a new technique worth trying in a certain population? Is an article worth discussing with colleagues? Deborah and her colleagues are not advancing the nursing profession through knowledge development by dismissing every article they have ever read as useless. Relying on skills learned years ago is not acceptable in today's practice environments where advances in technology and standards of practice are constantly being achieved.

What can the manager and the new CNS do to improve the staff's advancement of the nursing profession through active contributions to knowledge development? First, they may start a journal club. The CNS could choose a relevant article and have a roundtable discussion once a month. Results of this discussion could be posted in a central location for all staff to see. While it may not be well received at first, repeated exposure to relevant journal articles and productive discussions of them may help staff realize the benefits of staying up-to-date on the latest skills. Second, the manager could address the lack of incentive to use newly learned skills and knowledge by recruiting Deborah to work with the CNS to develop a Feeding Preemies Tips guideline for the nursing staff. It should be noted that Deborah might have something to contribute to the nursing literature on feeding infants and that this might be a good point for motivation to begin researching the nursing literature, starting with the subject of feeding infants, and then nursing issues in general. A staff meeting to explore ways to engage the nurses in reviewing professional standards data and their relation to the quality of care might stimulate the staff's interest in learning about what constitutes state-of-the-art practice and could also serve to improve morale. The manager could act as an advocate for the nursing staff by appealing to the hospital administration regarding monetary support for attending regional conferences. The CNS could work to initiate research in the unit that utilizes the expertise already present while encouraging the nurses in a way that promotes respect for the value of knowledge development

Although the unit's mortality data do not imply that the nurses are providing substandard care, the facts should motivate them to consider whether their general complacency about the value of research has caused them to miss important new techniques or approaches that would have a tangible effect on patient care. Blame cannot be placed on any one individual, but the cumulative effect of indifference to advancement of the profession by the staff, the manager, and nursing vice president has the potential to cause real harm to patients. The actions of nurses in higher levels of administration are directly implicated when a culture of complacency and uninformed practice exists.

Summary

Provision 7 has evolved from a statement that identifies the nurse's obligation to contribute to the "ongoing development of the professional's body of knowledge" to a statement that acknowledges the interdependence of the different nursing roles, recognizes the reciprocal obligations of the nurse to the profession and vice versa, and gives credence to the multifaceted complexities of contemporary nursing. The current provision extends beyond the obligation to contribute to knowledge development alone and includes other activities that serve to advance the nursing profession within education, administration, and even civic life. In doing so, the Code of Ethics now recognizes that (a) knowledge development, education and administration are intertwined, (b) each area can make important contributions to nursing, and (c) not all nurses have an interest in knowledge development via research, but each individual nurse has special interests and talents that can and should be used to advance the nursing profession. Provision 7 is now relevant for all nursing roles and is applicable to all individual nurses.

This provision encourages individual nurses to use their own talents and interests to create the moral link between their personal life, their individual practice, and the nursing profession as a whole. Provision 7 does not obligate nurses to actively engage in education, administration, and knowledge development. In fact, it is seldom possible for an individual nurse to excel in all three areas. More often, nurses are drawn to one particular area and can make significant contributions in that area. Provision 7 welcomes the individuality of each nurse. The three interpretive statements discussed in this chapter highlight the multiple ways in which nurses can contribute to the advancement of the profession, whether through participation in health policy application and development, engagement in the refinement of professional standards, or through the development, dissemination, and adaptation of knowledge. In this way, individual nurses can fulfill their obligations to themselves while contributing to the advancement of this vital profession.

References

Aiken L.H., S.P. Clarke, R.B. Cheung, D.M. Sloane, and J.H. Silber. 2003. Educational levels of hospital nurses and surgical patient mortality. *Journal of the American Medical Association* 290(12): 1617–23.

American Association Critical Care Nursing Certification Corporation. 2007. The AACN Synergy Model for Patient Care. http://www.certcorp.org/certcorp/certcorp.nsf/vwdoc/ SynModel?opendocument.

American Nurses Association (ANA). 1999. The National Center for Nursing Quality Indicators. http://www.nursingworld.org/quality/database.htm.

American Nurses Credentialing Center (ANCC). 2007. What Is the Magnet Recognition Program? http://nursecredentialing.org/magnet/.

Freidson, E. 1988. *Professional Powers: A Study of the Institutionalization of Formal Knowledge.* Chicago: University of Chicago Press.

Greenwood, E. 1957. Attributes of a profession. *Social Work* 2(3), 45–55.

Joint Commission on Accreditation of Hospital Organizations. (JCAHO). 2007. National Patient Safety Goals. Available: http://www.jointcommission.org/PatientSafety/ NationalPatientSafetyGoals/.

Miller, B.K., D. Adams, and L. Beck. 1993. A behavioral inventory for professionalism in nursing. *Journal of Professional Nursing* (9), 290–95.

National Institute of Nursing Research. 2007. http://www.ninr.nih.gov/.

Pavalko, T.M. 1971. *Sociology of Occupations and Professions.* Itasca, IL: Peacock.

Pew Charitable Trusts. 2007. http://www.pewtrusts.com/.

RAND Corporation. 2007. Health and health care research area. http://www.rand.org/ research_areas/health/.

Robert Wood Johnson Foundation. 2007. Nursing interest area. http://www.rwjf. org/ portfolios/interestarea.jsp?iaid=137.

Roberts, J.I., and T.M. Group. 1995. *Feminism and Nursing: An Historical Perspective on Power, Status, and Political Activism in the Nursing Profession.* Bloomington, IN: Indiana University Press.

Rogers, A.E., W. Hwang, L.D. Scott, L.H. Aiken, and D.F. Dinges. 2004. The working hours of hospital staff nurses and patient safety: Both errors and near errors are more likely to occur when hospital staff nurses work twelve or more hours at a stretch. *Health Affairs* 23(4): 202–212.

Rothschild, J.M., A.C. Hurley, C.P. Landrigan, J.W. Cronin, K. Martell-Waldrop, C. Foskett, E. Burdick, C.A. Czeisler, and D.W. Bates. 2006. Recovery from medical errors: the critical care nursing safety net. *Joint Commission Journal on Quality & Patient Safety* 32(2): 63–72.

About the Authors

Theresa S. Drought, PhD, RN, is currently an Assistant Professor at the University of Virginia School of Nursing. She has long been interested in the ethical issues related to professionalism in health care, serving as a nurse consultant to the California Medical Association's Council on Ethical Affairs, chair of the ANA\C Ethics Committee (ANA/California), and as a member of the American Nurses Association Task Force that produced the 2001 Code of Ethics for Nurses. Her publications and research address issues of professionalism and ethics in nursing and end-of-life decision making. Her current research focuses on decisions made by stranger surrogates. She received her PhD in nursing from the University of California at San Francisco in 2000.

Elizabeth G. Epstein, PhD, RN, received her PhD in Nursing from the University of Virginia in 2007. In August 2007, she took a position as Assistant Professor at the University of Virginia School of Nursing. Her doctoral dissertation and continuing interests are in ethics and end-of-life issues in the pediatric setting. In particular, she is interested in studying moral distress and moral obligations among healthcare providers, as well as determining how care-based ethics is evident in pediatric end-of-life care. She is a member of the American Society for Bioethics and Humanities. She serves as a facilitator for Conversations in Clinical Ethics, a multidisciplinary group at the University of Virginia that meets to discuss ethical issues that arise in the hospital setting.

Provision Eight

The nurse collaborates with other health professionals and the public in promoting community, national, and international efforts to meet health needs.

Provision Eight

Mary C. Silva, PhD, RN, FAAN

In the 16 years between the publication of the 1985 ANA *Code for Nurses with Interpretive Statements* and the publication of the 2001 ANA *Code of Ethics for Nurses with Interpretive Statements*, the world, its ethnicity, the healthcare system, the nursing profession, and the conceptualizations of ethics within nursing have changed mightily (Haidt et al, 2003; Manglitz, 2003). Advances in science and technology have increased globalization; cultural diversity in the United States and elsewhere has proliferated; new systems of care have altered how health care is delivered; nursing shortages have affected the profession; and approaches to ethics previously less visible (i.e., feminist, communitarian, and social ethics) have made their way into the nursing mainstream.

Although Provision 11 of the 1985 Code for Nurses and Provision 8 of the 2001 Code of Ethics sound similar, except for the addition of the word *international*, the interpretive statements of Provision 8 have changed substantially based on the factors noted above. Both interpretive statements mention nurses' commitment to meeting health needs; however, the 2001 Code clearly specifies that the nurse's commitment extends beyond specific individual patients' needs:

> The nurse has a responsibility to be aware not only of specific health needs of individual patients *but also of broader health concerns such as world hunger, environmental pollution, lack of access to heath care, violation of human rights, and inequitable distribution of nursing and healthcare resources* [italics added] (ANA, 2001; p. 23)

In addition, the 2001 Code also takes note of many of the causes of disease or trauma including *"barriers to health, such as poverty, homelessness, unsafe living conditions, abuse and violence, and lack of access to health services"* [italics added] (p. 24). With the exception of access to health care, none of these barriers were specified in the 1985 interpretive statement for this provision.

The interpretive statements in this revision also address another important concept that was omitted in the 1985 Code: cultural diversity and the nurse's responsibility to respond to it. According to Provision 8 of the 2001 Code:

The nurse also recognizes that health care is provided to culturally diverse populations in this country and in all parts of the world. In providing care, the nurse should avoid imposition of the nurse's own cultural values upon others. The nurse should affirm human dignity and show respect for the values and practices associated with different cultures and use approaches to care that reflect awareness and sensitivity (ANA, 2001; p. 24).

Clearly the world has changed and nursing's awareness of the moral dimensions of those changes is reflected in this revision of the Code.

Major Ethical Tenets Underlying Provision 8

The current literature contains many books and articles, both theoretical and applied, related to ethical tenets (Baily, 2003; Bodenheimer, 2003; Diekelmann, 2002; Veatch, 2003) and to the relationship between ethics and public health (Callahan and Jennings, 2002; Levin and Fleischman, 2002; Oberle and Tenove, 2000). Nurses, however, are most familiar and comfortable with ethical principles as set forth by Beauchamp and Childress (2001). In fact, the principle of respect for persons as well as the principles of autonomy, beneficence, nonmaleficence, justice, truth telling, promise keeping, and confidentiality formed the ethical bases for the 1985 Code. To these principles, nursing ethics are now concerned with other approaches, including a variety of critical social theories, such as critical (Frankfurt School), postcolonial, feminist, and communitarian social ethical theories, which are reflected in this revision of the Code.

Feminist Ethics

For many reasons, nurses have been reluctant to embrace feminism and its ethics. One reason may be a lack of self-awareness of the biases that are adopted by nurses from dominant culture or even the medical system itself. These are biases that may perpetuate social injustices rooted in gender, racial, or class distinctions. Another reason may be the negative stereotypes that extremists have unfortunately given to all forms of feminism.

Feminists (who may be women *or* men) are concerned about the barriers that close doors and, thus, systematically discriminate against or devalue women as a group. Many feminists are also concerned about systematic discrimination against men. Thus, the goal of feminism for many proponents is to examine the societal values and structures that cause oppression primarily to women, but also to men on the basis of gender, and to take constructive social action against them in order to promote better relationships between women and men and contribute to a more just society.

The shift from feminism to feminist ethics is almost seamless. According to Volbrecht: "Feminist ethics strives for social transformation that will empower all people to live freer, fuller lives" (2002, p. 162). Obviously, the societal factors listed in the new interpretive statement, such as world hunger, cultural imposition, lack of access to health care, human rights violations, homelessness, poverty, and violence, do *not* empower "all people to live freer, fuller lives." Each of the preceding factors represent ethical, feminist, and nursing concerns.

Feminist ethics also focuses on the belief that the voices of women should be heard and be given due weight in any theoretical formulations or practical application of ethics. Perhaps the best known work about these voices was penned by Carol Gilligan (1982). Gilligan wrote about a theme that women's voices address, one of responsibility for and a connection to others sustained through caring relationships.

This so-called ethics of care has had a profound influence on ethical thinking in nursing. Nurse proponents view *caring* as the essence of the ethical ideal of nursing. Although most often applied to individual, family, and small group relationships, one also can apply the concept of caring to the social concerns expressed in Provision 8. Although most nurses would agree that caring about patients is important, some nurses would not consider caring the essence of nursing. The reasons for this include: (a) nursing is not the only profession that cares, and (b) caring is not viewed as an empowering concept by persons in powerful positions that influence healthcare priorities and practice.

Communitarianism

Until recently, individualism dominated ethics in most of the Western world, particularly in the United States. This individualism can be seen in the priority given the ethical principle of respect for autonomy and individual rights. However, within the past three decades, there has emerged a movement away from an excessive focus on what is good for the individual to a more balanced emphasis on what is good for the community as well. According to Beauchamp and Childress, communitarians believe that "everything fundamental in ethics derives from communal values, the common good, social goals, traditional practices, and cooperative virtues" (2001, p. 362). In other words, the good of the community—whether one's local community or the world community—takes precedence over the good of the individual, whether embodied by personal rights or individual autonomy. Some communitarians, however, take a more moderate stance in that they believe that the good of the community and personal rights and individual autonomy should both be considered to ensure checks and balances against the excesses of either. In keeping with the preceding stance, Provision 8, with its emphasis on "promoting community, national, and international efforts to meet health needs" (ANA, 2001; p. 23) takes note of individuals' health needs, but emphasizes broader health needs that transcend individuals and affect the world community (e.g., hunger, poverty, violence).

Social Ethics

For many scholars, social ethics is grounded in the discipline of sociology. Here is what two medical sociologists have to say:

> We believe that sociology provides the most direct answer to the question, "Why bioethics?" The critical, relativizing stance of sociology allows us to see bioethics in the sweep of history and the context of medicine [health care] and society. A sociological approach lifts bioethics out of its clinical setting, examining the way it defines and solves ethical problems, the modes of reasoning it employs, and its influence on medical [health care] practice. (DeVries and Subedi, 1998; p. xiii).

Whereas much of traditional bioethics has had a more narrow focus (e.g., on clinical ethical issues), social ethics focuses on the "social bases of morality" (DeVries and Subedi, 1998; p. xiv). It applies such concepts as race, culture, roles, norms, customs, class, social institutions, and power to the social construction of moral issues within "the economic, political, religious, and institutional forces of a given historical period" (Light and McGee, 1998; p. 9).

This broad view of moral issues is integral to Provision 8. Nurses cannot holistically understand the moral issues inherent in such global healthcare problems as hunger, poverty, and violence without a strong grasp of the social forces that contribute to these problems. Herein nurses have an advantage; they are educated to understand and apply sociocultural and ethical concepts in their practice. Provision 9 emphasizes nursing's role in social ethics through its professional associations.

In summary, in order for readers to better understand the ethical tenets underlying Provision 8, three interrelated perspectives were briefly discussed: feminist ethics, communitarianism, and social ethics. What all three perspectives have in common is a focus on ethics that incorporates a larger societal picture of what constitutes morality.

Research on Ethical Issues Related to Provision 8

Public and global health nursing and the research conducted in these specialties are intrinsically related to this provision. Oberle and Tenove analyzed data from Canadian public health nurses, looking for ethical themes that could be found throughout their interviews. The five themes that emerged were as follows: (a) "relationships with healthcare professionals; (b) systems issues, such as staffing patterns; (c) character of relationships, such as knowing patients more broadly in smaller communities; (d) respect for persons, including being nonjudgmental; [and] (e) putting self at risk" (Oberle and Tenore, 2000; p. 428). The authors concluded by saying that there are many ethical concerns in public health nursing and that a systems approach supportive of ethical practice is necessary. The themes that they uncovered correlate well with several concepts in Provision 8: need "for interdisciplinary planning and collaborative partnerships among health professionals " (p. 23); "promoting health, welfare, and safety of all people" (p. 23); "support of and participation in community organizations and groups" (p. 24); and "health care is provided to culturally diverse populations" (ANA, 2001; p. 24).

The conclusions of this study support the research of Cooper and colleagues (2003). Theirs was an administrative ethics study conducted in the United States. The purpose of the study was to identify the ethical helps and challenges that managerial nurse leaders encounter in practice.

The three highest ranked ethical helps were: (a) "Your own personal moral values and standards" (p. 18), (b) "The fact that your immediate boss does not pressure you into compromising your ethical standards" (p. 18), and "An organizational environment/culture that does not encourage you to compromise your ethical values to achieve organizational goals" (p. 18). These ethical helps are based on the nurse's management style and an organizational culture that values ethics. In such environments, nurses are free to commit themselves to Provision 8's goal of "promoting the health, welfare, and safety of all people" (ANA, 2001; p. 23).

The result ranked first for ethical challenges was "intense competition in the healthcare industry which forces owners, managers, and supervisors to focus on the bottom line and not on ethics" (Cooper et al., 2003; p. 20). Other challenges (ranked 2 through 20) constituted less than 52% of the respondents' replies. The effects of negative social values and structure related to ethics would make it difficult for tenets of Provision 8 to be implemented.

Theory and Application Related to Public Health, Violence, and Ethics

Theory

According to Provision 8 "… the nurse supports initiatives to address barriers to health … such as… abuse and violence" (ANA, 2001; p. 24). Abuse and violence in health care have been addressed by many authors (e.g., Berman, 2003; Diekelmann, 2002; Lee and Saeed, 2001; Mercy et al, 2003; Volbrecht, 2002) and is viewed as a form of oppression. Oppression is the use of power in an unjust manner and is often a catalyst for violence. Violence is a type of oppression that is a threat to mental, physical, social, economic, or spiritual health. It can occur at the individual, family, community, or societal levels. Violence can be vertical, which means it can be perpetrated by groups among themselves. It is blind to gender, income, race, class, age, institutions, political viewpoints, or culture.

Violence is a health problem and, when focused on populations, a public or even global threat. According to Interpretive Statement 8.2, violence presents "existing threats to health and safety" (ANA, 2001; p. 24) of a community. Violence needs to be understood broadly. According to Diekelmann: "power, violence, and oppression accompany, although inadvertently, some of the 'best practices' of health care" (2002, p. xviii). For example, the emphasis on cure in health care that uses the best that science and technology have to offer may do profound physical, psychological, economic, and spiritual violence to those persons who cannot be cured. We call this "harming patients in the name of quality of life" (Fletcher et al., 2002; p. 3). The phrase also can be applied to nurses, communities, or cultures.

Application

Application of Provision 8 of the 2001 Code has been documented by Lee and Saeed (2001) in their article entitled "Oppression and Horizontal Violence: The Case of Nurses in Pakistan." After an excellent overview of forms of oppression, the authors discuss the following characteristics of oppressed groups as identified by Kaiser (1990): (a) harming of human dignity, (b) feeling hopeless and powerless, (c) internalizing lies and stereotypes, (d) infighting, and (e) engaging in horizontal violence where members of an oppressed group do violence to other members of the same oppressed group. Though this particular study focused on Pakistani nurses, horizontal violence occurs among nurses worldwide, in both developed and developing countries.

When Lee and Saeed focused on oppression and violence in Pakistan, especially as it relates to women and nurses, the four categories of assessment that they developed are relevant to the assessment of oppression and violence in any country worldwide.

- **Historical**—Is there evidence that oppression is present and has roots in history? Are there events in a group's past that have legitimized the oppression they experience?

- **Cultural**—Are there cultural taboos that marginalize a group? Are certain groups restricted in their participation in society?

- **Political**—Is the political system democratic and wholly egalitarian, or are equality and social justice only for select groups? Does the political system protect all groups from various forms of oppression, or are there laws that are oppressive in nature for particular groups?

- **Economic**—Are there classes that, due to low socioeconomic status, are oppressed? Are there groups that are privileged as a result of their economic status? (Lee and Saeed, 2001; pp. 19–21)

From these dimensions of assessment, they recommended the following strategies to reduce oppression and to empower nurses as professionals and providers of health care:

- Organize alliance-building groups to critically analyze the roots and forms of... oppression.

- Group analysis and problem solving to develop strategies that will eliminate the unequal power bases that exist.

- Authentic dialogue between nurses and their primary oppressor groups to examine circumstances in which nurses live and work, and assist group members to unlearn misinformation and oppressive behaviors.

- Develop unity within the groups so that power from within and power without can be used to challenge the status quo.

- Reconceptualize power and use of these new concepts in nursing practice, education, and research.

- Organize nurses into alliances to participate in health-policy planning.

- Develop position papers regarding the quality of basic and advanced nursing education or nursing work life.

- Develop proposals for additional budget allocations to nursing.

- Assisting in developing 5-year health plans for... [one's] country.

- Conduct research to define issues and concerns. Research such as determining exact numbers and describing the health workforce in... [one's] country is one example.

- Develop a media campaign to educate the public regarding the nursing profession; address the negative images and stereotypes that predominate, expose the origins of these images, and stress nurses' unique contribution to health care. (Lee and Saeed, 2001; p. 23)

How might feminist, communitarianism, and social ethics further inform these recommendations regarding nurse-to-nurse violence and its environment? How do these recommendations reflect the Code of Ethics—or not? What moral guidance can be drawn from the code that does or does not support these recommendations?

Theory and Application Related to Public Policy and Ethics

Theory

According to Interpretive Statement 8.2, "the nurse... participates in institutional and legislative efforts to promote health and meet national health objective" (ANA, 2001; p. 24). Institutional and legislative efforts to promote health through public policy and ethics (both explicitly and implied) have been addressed by many authors (American Public Health Association, 2002; Milo, 2002; Milstead, 2003; Shapiro, 1999; Silva, 2002; Tett et al, 2003). According to Shapiro:

The relationship between bioethics and [healthcare] public policy has become a rather broad subject that asks a rather simple question; namely, which moral imperatives that arise out of the study and consideration of bioethical issues should be reflected in [healthcare] public policies that govern us all. (Shapiro, 1999; p. 209)

Although the question is rather simple, the answers are more complex because of a lack of moral consensus on many healthcare ethical issues. This lack of moral consensus is partly due to social, cultural, legislative, economic, political, religious, and institutional diversity in the United States and elsewhere in the world. Nurses can choose to focus on what divides us or what unites us. Some nurses, however, choose to focus on what unites us.

Weston (2002) chooses to focus on what unites nurses. Here are some of his thoughts:

- For one thing, the diversity of values is probably overrated. Sometimes values appear to vary just because we have different beliefs about the facts (p. 8).

- Whether values are 'relative' or not, there is no way out of some good hard thinking (p. 10).

- Struggle and uncertainty are part of ethics, as they are part of life (p. 5).

- Rules can't replace thinking (p. 25).

- Whether we admit it or not, we do make our own [moral] decisions.... Choosing is inescapable (p. 28).

Weston's thoughts give pause to nurses and other healthcare professionals who are involved in "institutional and legislative efforts to promote health" (ANA, 2001, Provision 8; p. 24) through public policy that incorporates diversity.

Application

The application of Provision 8 has been documented by Sikma and Young in their 2003 article entitled "Nurse Delegation in Washington State: A Case Study of Concurrent Policy Implementation and Evaluation." Policy implementation and evaluation are congruent with the applied core functions of public and global health nursing. In addition, the Sikma and Young article fulfills the following tenet of Provision 8 of the 2001 Code: "The availability and accessibility of high quality health services to all people require both interdisciplinary planning and collaborative partnerships among health professionals and others at the community, national, and international levels" (ANA, 2001; p. 23). In this particular case study, the focus is at the community level.

According to Sikma and Young, the impetus for change regarding registered nurses' delegation of tasks to assistive personnel caring for disabled and older individuals in their homes was the result of "both the evolving nature of societal needs and values and the related dynamic changes in community health nursing practice" (Sikma and Young, 2003; pp. 53–54). The authors made clear that such changes and the evaluation and research associated with them could not have occurred by themselves; instead, ongoing interdisciplinary planning and collaborative partnerships were needed among special interest groups, public stakeholders, and the state of Washington.

The fact that policy implementation and health policy evaluation occurred concurrently made the research conducted by the authors more difficult because the preceding three stakeholder groups were involved with the research. Some of the special interest groups included professional organizations and nursing unions. Public stakeholders included senior and disability advocacy groups, as well as the general public. The State of Washington's involvement included senators and representatives, along with their staffs, as well as a variety of state analysts and others associated with health, elder, disability, quality control, and regulation and licensing services. In all, a total of 54 stakeholders were involved, including a joint House-Senate oversight committee to endorse the evaluation research plan and monitor the study's progress.

Some of the concerns of the stakeholders included preserving and respecting autonomy for seniors and disabled persons, ensuring safety of those clients, and safeguarding the scope of nursing practice. Other concerns involved adequate education of the caregiver staff and regulatory and reimbursement issues. In addition, special interest stakeholders had so many concerns about the policy research expertise of the authors and of the study design that the stakeholders requested their own expert to evaluate the soundness of the evaluation study. Fortunately, the study was deemed sound, but the authors had to employ several strategies to ensure stakeholder credibility.

The strategies employed by the authors (Sikma and Young, 2003) included the following: (a) "identifying stakeholders and their agendas" (p. 57); (b) "translating research designs and methods" (p. 57); (c) "working through the politics of the group" (p. 58); (d) "ongoing communication with stakeholders" (p. 59); and (e) "dissemination of results to multiple audiences" (p. 59). The authors concluded by saying:

> This case study illustrates the complexities of collaboration in policy evaluation research and highlights an effective partnership between researchers, policy makers, providers, and consumers in shaping legislation that addresses multiple goals (Sikma and Young, 2003; p. 60).

The legislation shaped was entitled An Act Relating to Long-Term Care. The goals accomplished were a practice change in the State of Washington's legislation

regarding community health registered nurses' task delegation to assistive personnel caring for elders and persons with disabilities in their homes and a concurrent,
rigorous policy evaluation of that change.

How might feminism, communitarianism, and social ethics inform, challenge, or
guide the strategies employed by these authors? What ethical principles are operative
in this project? What ethical principles might be in conflict? What are the values
that nursing would assert in this project? How might the Code of Ethics inform,
challenge, or guide this project and any that might arise from it?

Theory and Application Related to Culturally Diverse Populations and Ethics

Theory

Provision 8 emphasizes culturally diverse worldwide populations, respect for persons
and their ways of life, and cultural values, imposition, sensitivity, and competence.
The concepts of cultural diversity and competence as they relate to health care have
been addressed by many authors (Campinha-Bacote, 2003; Chaffee, 2002; Pratt,
2002), although the relationships among the preceding four concepts and ethics
tend to be implicit. Other authors have helped to close the gap between culture
and ethics by making the relationship between them more explicit (Bennett et al.,
2003; Haidt et al, 2003; Pang et al., 2003). Nurses are already familiar with the
concepts that underlie culture such as customs, beliefs, values, norms, and so forth
that are learned, widely shared, and transmitted from generation to generation
within a certain social group. Nurses attuned to cultural diversity recognize and
appreciate the differences between and among these social groups. Although many
definitions of cultural diversity exist, the more expansive ones are more in keeping
with the spirit of Provision 8 of the 2001 Code and include race, socioeconomic and
occupational status, religious affiliation, political orientation, physical size, gender,
age, and language.

Of these factors, one in the current literature that has received considerable
attention is race (Baldwin, 2003; Manglitz, 2003; Treadwell and Ro, 2003). Overall,
the major concern expressed in this literature is that race affects the nature of
health problems and the quality of healthcare that one receives. Baldwin discusses
how some races have an increased likelihood of cancer, diabetes, HIV/AIDS, and
cerebrovascular and cardiovascular diseases. In addition, many culturally diverse
persons in the United State are blamed for their poor health and their reluctance
to use the predominant white healthcare system. Why? Because, according to

Manglitz being "White in America" constitutes a historical and social-cultural construction of privilege that usually goes unrecognized by whites, but not by people of color. Manglitz continues: "We need to develop ways to rearticulate a way to be White without dominating and subjugating people in the process" (Manglitz, 2003; p. 131). Although race was highlighted here as an example, any of the faces of cultural diversity could address the concept of privilege (e.g., gender, age, occupational status) that is capable of oppression of other persons, groups, or societies. A characteristic of privileged groups is that they impose their cultural values on others. Provision 8 of the 2001 Code clearly states that cultural imposition should be avoided. And yet, as indicated above, the unrecognized imposition of culture and its norms is an enormous impediment to correcting health disparities and other social injustices.

Application

Provision 8 also states that nurses should "show respect for the values and practices associated with different cultures and use approaches to care that reflect awareness and sensitivity" (ANA, 2001; p. 24). Two approaches nurses can use that are in keeping with this Provision are careful listening to clients' stories about cultural diversity and use of sensitive assessment tools to help ensure cultural awareness.

The nurse's careful listening to clients' stories about cultural diversity is a type of caring practice that helps to reveal the ethics embedded within the stories. Let's listen to a true story of a Saudi Arabian doctoral nursing student studying in the United States:

> For my internship, I was placed in a senior retirement center. I was sitting in a meeting with the American daughter and son of potential new residents. The daughter was very excited; she was telling me a story about how they finally convinced their parents to sell their home and belongings so that they could move into a retirement center. The daughter's mood was exuberant and she was smiling. She turned to me and said, "Isn't this wonderful?" I was totally shocked and I knew that my face revealed horror. In my country parents would never be asked to sell their homes or possessions. No one would speak to me if I did such a thing to my parents. I cried all the way home (Anonymous).

The preceding story is interesting because it offers an opportunity to see how a person from another culture views an increasingly acceptable norm in American society—the placing of elderly parents into senior retirement centers. This scenario raised no ethical concerns for the daughter and son, but was clearly a violation of the ethical principle of respect for persons, or, more specifically, respect for parents and elders, in the Saudi culture. Although difficult, the student eventually was able to accept the American daughter and son's decision because she recognized the need to respond to others in light of their cultural values and norms and not her own. In addition to sensitive, discerning listening, Chaffee offers some good, yet simple and cost-effective, advice: "In today's 'global village,' there is one universally recognized gesture: the smile" (2002, p. 98).

In reviewing the preceding information related to culturally diverse populations and ethics, the reader is challenged to apply feminist ethics, communitarianism, and social ethics to the issues of race, ethnicity, and cultural diversity in our healthcare system. What values, priorities and cultural norms have you embraced that need to be "uncovered"? Where did you learn them? Do they conflict with nursing values as articulated in the Code of Ethics, the Social Policy Statement, and other ANA documents? What values, priorities, and cultural norms has American nursing embraced that need to be "uncovered"? How are these norms made manifest? How would feminism, communitarian, and social ethics assess our profession's norms?

Implications of Provision 8

Implications of Provision 8 of the 2001 Code of Ethics for Nurses with Interpretive Statements are as follows:

- Nurses need to expand their understanding of major ethical tenets underlying Provision 8: feminist ethics, communitarianism, and social ethics. These are less familiar to nurses than are classic ethical theories and principles. Yet, Provision 8 deals with health needs and nurses' responsibilities to the world community; thus, ethical tenets that incorporate a global viewpoint are needed to ensure a healthy world and its environment.

- Because Provision 8 focuses on global health concerns (e.g., world hunger, environmental pollution, inequitable health care, homelessness, poverty) that have profound implications for the world's health, nurses must be well prepared to incorporate and apply public health knowledge to their practice. This knowledge must be progressive to meet not only known health concerns and threats, but those of the future as well.

- Provision 8 states that a responsibility of the nurse is to participate in legislative efforts related to health. Nurses must continue to be involved in public policy initiatives that promote the public good. Nurses must also recognize that ethics is the foundation for the public good.

- Provision 8's focus on respect for cultural diversity is essential in a heterogeneous country like the United States. Many of our country's ills, as well as those of the world, are due to an attitude of privilege or even imperialism toward other people. This trait breeds alienation that profoundly affects the quality of health care of those persons, communities, or societies who feel that they are treated as second-class citizens. Provision 8 of the 2001 Code of Ethics for Nurses clearly states that the nurse has an ethical obligation to be aware of and sensitive to diversity. The nursing profession and individual nurses must act on this obligation regardless of the nurse's role or work setting.

- Increased research related to ethics is needed on health needs, concerns, and the nurse's responsibilities to the public discussed in Provision 8.

If nurses take to heart all of the ethical tenets, concepts, and implications embedded in Provision 8 of the 2001 Code, they will be moved to "collaborate with other health professionals and the public in promoting community, national, and international efforts to meet health needs" (ANA, 2001; p. 4).

References

All online references were accessed in December 2007.

American Nurses Association. 1985. *Code for Nurses with Interpretive Statements*. Kansas City, MO: ANA.

American Nurses Association. 2001. *Code of Ethics for Nurses with Interpretive Statements*. Washington, DC: American Nurses Publishing.

American Public Health Association. 2002. Policy statements adopted by the Governing Council of the American Public Health Association, October 24, 2001. *American Journal of Public Health* 92: 451–83.

Baily, M.A. 2003. Managed care organizations and the rationing problem. *Hastings Center Report* 33(1): 34–42.

Baldwin, D.M. 2003. Disparities in health and health care: Focusing efforts to eliminate unequal burdens. *Online Journal of Issues in Nursing* 8(1; January 31): Article 1. http:// www.nursingworld.org/ojin/topic20/tpc20_1.html.

Beauchamp, T.L., and J.F. Childress. 2001. *Principles of Biomedical Ethics*, 5th ed. New York: Oxford University Press.

Bennett, J.A., M.L. Fleming, L. Mackin, A. Hughes, M. Wallhagen, and J. Kayser-Jones. 2003. Recruiting ethnically diverse nurses to graduate education in gerontological nursing: Lessons from a successful program. *Journal of Gerontological Nursing* 29(3): 17–22.

Berman, H. 2003. Getting critical with children: Empowering approaches with a disempowered group. *Advances in Nursing Science* 26(2): 102–13.

Bodenheimer, T. 2003. The movement for universal health insurance: Finding common ground. *American Journal of Public Health* 93: 112–15.

Callahan, D., and B. Jennings. 2002. Ethics and public health: Forging a strong relationship. *American Journal of Public Health* 92: 169–76.

Campinha-Bacote, J. 2002. Cultural competence in psychiatric nursing: Have you "ASKED" the right questions? *Journal of the American Psychiatric Association* 8(16): 183–87.

Campinha-Bacote, J. 2003. Many faces: Addressing diversity in health care. *Online Journal of Issues in Nursing* 8 (1; January 31): Article 2. http://www.nursingworld.org/ojin/topic20/ tpc20_2.html.

Chaffee, M.W. 2002. Communication skills for political success. In *Policy and Politics in Nursing and Health Care*, 4th ed., 93–107. St. Louis, MO: Saunders.

Cooper, R.W., G.L. Frank, C.A. Gouty, and M.M. Hansen. 2003. Ethical helps and challenges faced by nurse leaders in the healthcare industry. *Journal of Nursing Administration* 33(1): 17–23.

DeVries, R., and J. Subedi, eds. 1998. *Bioethics and Society: Constructing the Ethical Enterprise.* Upper Saddle River, NJ: Prentice Hall.

Diekelmann, N.L., ed. 2002. *First Do No Harm: Power, Oppression, and Violence in Healthcare.* Madison, WI: The University of Wisconsin Press.

Fletcher, J.J., M.C. Silva, and J.M. Sorrell. 2002. Harming patients in the name of quality of life. In *First, Do No Harm: Power, Oppression, and Violence in Healthcare*, pp. 3–48. Madison, WI: The University of Wisconsin Press.

Gilligan, C. 1982. *In a Different Voice: Psychological Theory and Women's Development.* Cambridge, MA: Harvard University Press.

Haidt, J., E. Rosenberg, and H. Hom. 2003. Differentiating diversities: Moral diversity is not like other kinds. *Journal of Applied Social Psychology* 33(1): 1–36.

Guide to the Code of Ethics for Nurses

Kaiser, S. 1990. Issues of culture and oppression in organizations. http://www. bizgrowth. com/html.

Lee, M.B., and I. Saeed. 2001. Oppression and horizontal violence: The case of nurses in Pakistan. *Nursing Forum* 36(1): 15–24.

Levin, B.W., and A.R. Fleischman. 2002. Public health and bioethics: The benefits of collaboration. *American Journal of Public Health* 92: 165–67.

Light, D.W., and G. McGee. 1998. On the social embeddedness of bioethics. In *Bioethics and Society: Constructing the Ethical Enterprise*, pp. 1–15. Upper Saddle River, NJ: Prentice Hall.

Manglitz, E. 2003. Challenging White privilege in adult education: A critical review of the literature. *Adult Education Quarterly* 53(2): 119–34.

Mercy, J.A., E.G. Krug, L.L. Dahlberg, and A.B. Zwi. 2003. Violence and health: The United States in a global perspective. *American Journal of Public Health* 92: 256–61.

Milio, N. 2002. Where policy hits the pavement: Contemporary issues in communities. In *Policy and Politics in Nursing and Health Care*, 4th ed., pp. 659–68. St. Louis, MO: Saunders.

Milstead, J.A. 2003. Interweaving policy and diversity. *Online Journal of Issues in Nursing* 8(1; January 31): Article 4. http://www.nursingworld.org/ojin/topic20/tpc20_4html.

Oberle, K., and S. Tenove. 2000. Ethical issues in public health nursing. *Nursing Ethics* 7: 425–38.

Pang, S.M., A. Sawada, E. Konishi, D.P. Olsen, P.L. Yu, M.F. Chan, and N. Mayum. 2003. A comparative study of Chinese, American, and Japanese nurses' perceptions of ethical role responsibilities. *Nursing Ethics* 10(3): 295–311.

Pratt, G. 2002. Collaborating across our differences. *Gender, Place and Culture* 9(2): 195–200.

Shapiro, H.T. 1999. Reflections on the interface of bioethics, public policy, and science. *Kennedy Institute of Ethics Journal* 9(3): 209–24.

Sikma, S.K., and H.M. Young. 2003. Nurse delegation in Washington State: A case study of concurrent policy implementation and evaluation. *Policy, Politics, & Nursing Practice* 4(1): 53–61.

Silva, M.C. 2002. Ethical issues in health care, public policy, and politics. In *Policy and Politics in Nursing and Health Care*, 4th ed., 177–84. St. Louis, MO: Saunders.

Tett, L., J. Crowther, and P. O'Hara. 2003. Collaborative partnerships in commumunity education. *Journal of Educational Policy* 18(1): 37–51.

Treadwell, H.M., and M. Ro. 2003. Poverty, race, and the invisible men. *American Journal of Public Health* 93: 705–7.

Veatch, R.M. 2003. *The Basics of Bioethics*, 2nd ed. Upper Saddle River, NJ: Prentice Hall.

Volbrecht, R.M. 2002. *Nursing Ethics: Communities in Dialogue.* Upper Saddle River, NJ: Prentice Hall.

Weston, A. 2002. *A Practical Companion to Ethics*, 2nd ed. New York: Oxford University Press.

About the Author

Mary C. Silva, PhD, RN, FAAN, received her BSN and MS from the Ohio State University and her PhD from the University of Maryland. In addition, she undertook postdoctoral studies at Georgetown University. She has taught healthcare ethics at the master's and doctoral levels and published extensively in the area of ethics, beginning in the 1970s. She is currently Professor Emerita at George Mason University in Fairfax, Virginia. Dr. Silva is also a Fellow in the American Academy of Nursing.

Provision Nine

The profession of nursing, as represented by associations and their members, is responsible for articulating nursing values, for maintaining the integrity of the profession and its practice, and for shaping social policy.

Provision Nine

Marsha D.M. Fowler, PhD, MDiv, MS, RN, FAAN

Many of the elements of this provision are found in previous versions of the Code of Ethics, as will be shown shortly. However, the inclusion of a provision directed toward the profession through its associations, rather than toward the individual nurse, is dramatically new. The provisions of all previous Codes have been directed toward individual nurses, most often the nurse at the bedside. In the later revisions, some attention was given to nurse researchers, and then, in the most recent Codes, to nurse educators as well. The 2001 Code expands to include all nurses in all nursing positions, as well as the profession itself. This shift in the Code reflects the ongoing shift in U.S. nursing practice, much as earlier Codes reflected their time. For instance, earliest modern nursing, after the Civil War, took place in the home as "private duty nursing," in which nurses were hired by the family. Private duty nursing dominated nursing practice until World War II, after which the majority of nursing shifted from the home to the hospital and nurses became employees of the hospital, known as "general duty" nursing. Prior to this shift, hospitals were largely staffed by students. Even into the 1970s, there was a remnant of private duty nursing, often called "specialing," within hospitals. Private duty nursing within the hospital context rapidly disappears after the late 1960s with the advent of the centralization of illness care, the inception of intensive care units, and the subsequent specialization and subspecialization within nursing.

The effect that the location of nursing in the home had upon codes of ethics was that they were written for a nurse who did not receive direct supervision and who had to make clinical and moral decisions on her (mostly) own. *Confidentiality* received particularly heavy emphasis as the nurse was in a position to observe the goings-on within a family home. In this early period, many nursing educators were physicians, though a nurse was often the "superintendent" of the nursing school. The shift toward nurses as nurse educators was slow in coming, accelerating after WWII, and reaching completion by the 1970s. As for research, the role of a nurse researcher did not rise until well after the 1950s. Thus, early codes would not have "needed" to address nurse educators or nurse researchers, or, of course, nurse practitioners or nurses in nonstandard positions. This Code, then, departs from previous

Codes by including all nurses in all nursing positions individually and all nurses collectively through nursing associations. This provision goes farther and specifically focuses on the role of professional associations in social ethics.

Social ethics may be defined as the domain of ethics that deals with "issues of social order—the good, right, and ought in the organization of human communities and the shaping of social policies. Hence the subject matter of social ethics is moral rightness and goodness in the shaping of human society."[1] There are three major functions of social ethics, all of which fall within the legitimate, if not essential, sphere of the professional nursing association: reform of the profession, epidictic discourse (which is a type of public values-based speaking), and social reform.[2]

The first function of social ethics—reform of the profession—assures that the profession itself keeps its own house clean. Reform seeks to bring the profession and its practice, goals, and aspirations into conformity with the values that it holds dear. At times, this necessitates change within the professional community itself, seeking to move the profession toward an envisioned ideal, to bring the "ought" into conformity with the reality of the profession's lived expression. This aspect of social ethics demands an intentional, ongoing, critical self-reflection and self-evaluation of the profession based on a range of critical theories that can assist in an incisive, rigorous self-assessment of the profession.

"Epidictic discourse," the second function of social ethics, refers to a form of communication that takes place within and for the group. Unfortunately, *epidictic* has no synonym in the English language. Epidictic discourse refers to that kind of speech that reaffirms and reinforces the values that the community itself embraces, especially when they are confronted by competing values. It "sets out to increase the intensity of adherence to certain values, which might not be contested when considered on their own but may nevertheless not prevail against other values that might come into conflict with them."[3] Epidictic discourse is essentially a "rallying cry" that reinforces the group's values to and for the group. It strengthens the values that are held in common by the group and the speaker, thus "making use of dispositions already present in the audience."[4] Epidictic discourse galvanizes the group to employ the group's cherished values in order both to bring about the changes elicited by the first function of social ethics, and to move the group into the third function of social ethics—speaking the values of the group into society at large to help bring about social change that is congruent with the group's values.[5] Examples of epidictic speech in public address abound. A few examples include: Martin Luther King's "I Have a Dream"; John Kennedy's *"Ich bin ein Berliner"*; Franklin Roosevelt's Pearl Harbor address to the Nation; Douglas MacArthur's farewell address to Congress; Patrick Henry's "Give Me Liberty or Give Me Death." Epidictic discourse is not solely the domain of famous men. These women's speeches are excellent examples as well: Jane Addams' "The Subjective Necessity for Social Settlements"; Susan Anthony's "On Women's Right to Vote"; Eleanor Roosevelt's "The Struggle for Human Rights"; Sojourner Truth's "Ain't I a Woman?"; and Margaret Sanger's "The Children's Era."

The third aspect of social ethics is that of social reform. In this, the profession critiques society and attempts to bring about social change that is consistent with the values of the group. For instance, if the group affirms affordable, accessible health care for all, it would assess the current state of the healthcare system for cost, distribution, and fairness of costs; access and ease of access by all sectors of society, including those with limitations such as mobility, age, literacy, etc. and including ethnic and minority constituencies; and openness of the system to all, including resident noncitizens, tourists, and others. It is expected that all nurses will be involved in this aspect of the profession's social ethics. However, the actual implementation of social criticism and social change generally depends upon collective action, usually through a professional association. In order to engage in social criticism and to bring about social change, the profession must have knowledge based in theories that can guide and deepen social analysis and critique. Here we often see postcolonial, feminist, liberation, Marxist, or critical social theories employed, both to assess and critique society as well as the profession itself. (Note that these are the same theories that would be used to critique the profession itself.) In order to bring about social change, these theories and a knowledge of political and policy processes becomes essential. The resources of the professional association, including its political action committees, would then be drawn upon to support action for social change. It is important for this aspect of the profession's social ethics that nurse educators include in nursing curricula content on ethics relating to issues of justice, social theories, nursing history related to social involvement of nursing and nurses, health policy formulation, and the state and federal political process. These three functions of social ethics (reform within, epidictic discourse, and social reform) are incorporated into the first part of the interpretive statement Assertion of Values.

Interpretive Statement 9.1: Assertion of Values

All three functions of social ethics are incorporated, in brief, into this section. But why this provision? Why any concern for social ethics in a code of ethics for nursing?

Nursing ethics in the United States has always been intimately concerned with the shape of society and its affect upon health and illness, that is, with social ethics. The profession's historical and continuing involvement with working for the health of all is remarkable and it is the stuff of "pride of profession." This abiding concern for social ethics is reflected in early nursing ethics curricula. In 1917, the National League for Nursing Education (NLNE) established curricular requirements for ethics in nursing education within its Standard Curriculum for Schools of Nursing. The standard called for 10 hours of ethics instruction in the second year, a number of hours coequal to that of other major topics such as medical nursing. The basic lectures were to include content on ethical theory, personal ethics, professional ethics, clinically applied ethics, and social ethics.[6] Topics to be covered in the social ethics content included "the social virtues" and "ethical principles as applied to community life." State boards of registered nursing also specified curricular requirements in social ethics. The California State Board of Health's Bureau of Registration of Nurses 1916 curricular requirements in social ethics included: "democracy and social ethics," "modern industry," "housing reform," and "the spirit of youth and the city streets."[7]

Interpretive Statement 9.2: The Profession Carries Out Its Collective Responsibility through Professional Associations

The social ethics of a profession is most often, though not exclusively, exercised through its professional associations; that is, through collectives of nurses rather than by individual nurses themselves. As a part of keeping our own house, professional associations shepherd the creation and ongoing revision of such core materials as standards of practice, criteria for accreditation of nursing educational programs, certification processes, code of ethics, and social contract (such as ANA's Nursing's Social Policy Statement). Collectively, in nursing these are intended to produce a baseline of safe nursing practice as a measure of the profession's responsibility to society to evaluate its practice and practitioners. The Code of Ethics is a distinctive kind of professional standard as it establishes moral guidelines for members of the profession and it publicly states the values of the profession. The nursing profession, through its first and official spokes-organization, the American Nurses Association, has always viewed the Code as having the utmost importance.

The history of the Code begins with the meeting of delegates and representatives of the American Society of Superintendents of Training Schools for Nurses, who convened to establish a professional association for nurses. The Nurses' Associated Alumnae of the United States and Canada (later the ANA and the Canadian

Nurses' Associations, respectively) was formed and the articles of incorporation were written at that meeting. In the articles of incorporation, they identified their purposes, the first of which was "to establish and maintain a code of ethics."[8] Thus, establishing and maintaining a Code for the profession is the premier task of the Association. Two attempts to establish a Code (1926, 1940) failed before the Code for Professional Nurses was officially adopted by the ANA House of Delegates in 1950. Subsequent to its adoption, the Code has undergone revision approximately every 10 years in order to remain morally responsive to the context and setting of nursing. Some revisions have been minor, others have been major. With the inception of the inclusion of "interpretive statements," the provisions of the Code have remained the same over long periods of time, while the interpretive statements have undergone substantial revision. That first Code and its successive revisions publicly made explicit the moral "contract between the profession and society" as a part of the profession's overall accountability to society.

Interpretive Statement 9.3: Intraprofessional Integrity

This section of the provision's interpretive statements alludes to the fact that nursing (like all social structures) is comprised of "meaning and value structures," as well as "power structures." The meaning and value structures of a profession (as expressed by its representative group, the professional association) are those aspects of the nursing association that embody the ideals, values, and ethics of the profession. This would include not only the Code of Ethics and the Social Policy Statement, but also the ANA Center for Ethics and Human Rights, the moral policies and position statements published by the Association, its ethics committees, and so on. Meaning and value structures articulate the values, moral ideals, and moral requirements of a group, and also serve to inform and guide, critique—and sometimes to correct—the goals, practices, or activities of a profession. Meaning and value structures are juxtaposed against power structures, which are those social structures that embody, utilize, or direct power in any of its forms. Power comes in many forms, including politics, economics, social prestige, honor, respect, expertise, and authority. Power structures enable a group to achieve its goals. Without adequate meaning and value structures, power structures can exercise runaway self-interest. Without power structures, meaning and values structures are dead in the water. Meaning and value structures must work reciprocally with power structures to advance the goals of a group in accord with its ideals.[9]

To "encourage the professional organization and its members to function in accord with [its] values," the professional association is to "promote awareness of and adherence to the Code of Ethics and to critique the activities and ends of the professional association itself."[10] Awareness of the Code begins, properly, in early nursing education. Awareness is furthered by ANA's distribution of the Code "bookmarks," and other Code-related materials, and by posting the full text of the Code of Ethics with Interpretive Statements on the ANA website.[11] Promoting adherence to the Code has taken a number of forms. In the 1960s, the ANA actually formulated a document process and guidelines for reporting what were thought to be violations of the Code.[12] The Guidelines open with the quote: "Unfortunately, there are always those whose ethical practice is far less than acceptable. Yet a profession must assume responsibility for guaranteeing to the public that all services rendered by its members are of high quality."[13] This document was not subsequently revised and fell out of print. Today, adherence to the Code is generally fostered by "moral suasion;" that is, by persuasion and pressure for adherence to moral standards, which cannot be compelled or forced. The moral consequences of a proven violation of the Code are reprimand or censure by the organization or expulsion from membership. This does not necessarily affect a nurse's work-a-day world as the consequences are limited to the nurse's relationship with the professional association. However, moral violations will affect one's stature, respect, and honor among peers, and can affect self-respect.

The interpretive statement states that:

> Legitimate concerns for the self-interest of the association and the profession are balanced by a commitment to the social goods that are sought. Through critical self-reflection and self-evaluation, associations must foster change within themselves, seeking to move the professional community toward its stated ideals.[14]

Bundled up in the phrase "legitimate concerns for the self-interest of the association and the profession…" is a long history of concern for a just and equitable wage/salary for nurses. Previous Codes have emphasized "working conditions"[15] and "conditions of practice conducive to high quality nursing practice,"[16] as well as "the importance of working conditions to recruitment to nursing, and the social stature of the profession."[17] The more immediate and pressing concern underneath these statements, however, has been for just wages/salaries for nurses.

The Suggested Code of 1926 is rather more direct:

> Economic independence is admittedly one of the first duties of every citizen… Self-realization and the most complete development of individual capacities are the ideals of present-day society for all of its members. There is no ground for expecting the nurse to be an exception to this rule nor its corollary that self-development can best be nurtured in the soil of economic self-respect…

[but] no worker is welcome to the ranks of nursing who does not put the ideal of service above that of remuneration.[18]

The Tentative Code of 1940 makes statements that give an underlying view of some of the problems nurses faced:

In some instances, the economic status of the patient undoubtedly will command the gratuitous services of nurses; but the officers of endowed institutions or hospitals...have no claim upon the nurse for unremunerated services....If an institution organized to provide adequate service for the sick, including nursing care, for any reason cannot fulfill this obligation, it should not expect to commandeer the unremunerated, or markedly under-paid, services of nurses.[19]

This is a snapshot of a problem faced by nurses in the 1940s (and earlier). This, of course, does not happen today. Or does it? There is no moral difference between the picture given by the Tentative Code and institutions today that expect "the unremunerated, or markedly underpaid, services of nurses" by denying nurses "overtime" pay, while expecting overtime service. Provision 9 of the 1950 Code states: "the nurse has an obligation to give conscientious service and in return is entitled to just remuneration."[20] Indeed. However softened by the "work condi-tions" language in the 1960 Code and later versions, issues of just compensation, "economic self-respect," salary-compression, gender equity, work equivalency salaries, and a "savings plans which will bring her financial security in old age" still loom large for the nursing profession.

The interpretive statement also calls for "critical self-reflection and self-evalua-tion" of associations to "foster change within themselves, seeking to move the pro-fessional community toward its stated goals."[21] Historically, the American Nurses Association has been involved in self-reflection and social change.

In the late 1800s and early 1900s, when the United States engaged in the legal enslavement of racial minorities, women were legally defined as chattel and denied suffrage, and gender-based social roles were rigidly defined with the legal exclusion of women from some roles (e.g., physician); there were laws against teaching about or possessing contraceptives, little or no protection of children in sweat shops under labor laws, and no laws against domestic violence or animal cruelty. Eventually, American society came to address these ills in at least some modest measure, though remnants of some remain today, over 125 years later. The nursing association that formed 107 years ago has worked for the correction of some of these ills.

The Tentative Code states that "a truly professional nurse with broad social vision will have a sympathetic understanding of different creeds, nationalities, and races and in any case she will not permit her personal attitude toward these various groups to interfere with her function as a nurse."[22] In the adopted 1950 Code, it states in the preamble that: "Need for nursing is universal. Professional service is therefore unrestricted by considerations of nationality, race, creed, or color."[23] Successive codes reiterate this basic position and even enlarge it to encompass a wide range of other forms of social disadvantagement, stigma, prejudice, and oppression.

At one point, however, these statements were not in alignment with the current situation of society, which still permitted and, sometimes, legally authorized various organized social manifestations of prejudice. At that time, the professional association operated on a federated model where the parent organization did not have members, rather nurses were members of state nurses associations (SNAs) which simultaneously conferred American Nurses Association (ANA) membership. States established their own criteria for membership. Some of these constituent states had denied membership in the organization to those who were fully qualified, but were of African descent, in whole or in part. The Association could not control the state associations' criteria for membership. What ought the Association do? Alternatives were for the Association to ignore the situation and proceed as usual. It could have also changed its organizational structure, a massive undertaking, or revised the then current Code. What ought the Association to have done?

Nursing as a profession has long espoused a principal of egalitarianism, even when society openly permitted or even authorized a wide range of prejudicial "isms": racism, sexism, sectarianism, etc. This, of course, flew in the face of the societal reality of dramatic social inequalities. In a profession that has remained predominantly Anglo, Christian, and female, this persistent egalitarianism is somewhat unexpected. And yet, it is interesting to speculate, and fodder for research, that because nursing has remained female dominant, it identifies with social groups that, like women, have been socially disadvantaged. Therefore, with this commitment to equalitarianism, it posed a painful moral quandary for the American Nurses Association when some SNAs barred fully qualified black nurses from membership, thereby denying them ANA membership in the federated model. What ought a professional association do? In 1948, the American Nurses Association made provision for black nurses to have direct membership in ANA, without SNA membership. If an association proclaims that nurses should not discriminate on prejudicial grounds against those not of the dominant race, creed, color, or religion, it cannot sanction such discrimination within its own organization. The first task of social ethics is to clean one's own house, which is what the ANA did. As the 2001 Code puts it: "Through critical self-reflection and self-evaluation, associations must foster change within themselves, seeking to move the professional community toward its stated ideals."[24] The action of the 1948 ANA exemplified the values expressed in this provision, even though there was no such provision in the first Code for Professional Nurses in 1950.

Interpretive Statement 9.4: Social Reform

Nursing's history is rich with examples of nurses who have, individually, brought about social–moral change. Many of the early women, and some men, counted as nurses, actually preceded the establishment of nursing schools in the United States. Even so, their achievements are credited to nursing. These include Dorothea Lynde Dix, Walt Whitman, Clara Harlowe Barton, Araminta (Harriet) Ross Tubman, Capt. Sally Tompkins, and Mary Ann Ball Bickerdyke, among others. Of the women who received formal nursing education, three historic figures will serve as examples of individuals who, by themselves, wrought social change.

- **Margaret Higgins Sanger** was shocked that women were unable to obtain accurate and effective birth control, which she believed was foundational to the freedom and independence of women. She challenged the 1873 Federal Comstock law that banned the dissemination of contraceptive information. She published a monthly paper, *The Woman Rebel*, in which she advocated for women's right to use contraception. She was indicted for violating postal obscenity laws, jumped bail, and escaped to England. Subsequently, she worked tirelessly in England and then again in the United States for women's rights to contraceptive information and contraceptives.[25]

- **Lillian D. Wald** was asked to organize a nursing program to meet the needs of the impoverished immigrant population of Manhattan in the late 19th century. She observed the terrible conditions under which the city's poor survived. Wald was deeply moved and decided to dedicate her life to providing health and social services to the city's poor. In 1893, with Mary Brewster, she established The Henry Street Settlement, which eventually became the Visiting Nurse Service of New York City. Wald pioneered the creation of public health nursing, visiting nursing, and the social service system. By 1916, the Settlement had 250 nurses and offered health care, housing, education, employment assistance, and recreational activities to thousands of the city's poor families and individuals.

- **Isabel Adams Hampton Robb** served as Superintendent at the Illinois Training School in the Cook County Hospital; then became the first superintendent of the new nursing school at Johns Hopkins Hospital in Baltimore. After her marriage, she became a professor of gynecology at Case Western Reserve University. She brought about major changes in the process and curriculum of nursing education. Robb organized a nursing section at the International Congress of Charities, Corrections and Philanthropy of the World Columbian Exposition held in Chicago. The section became the first nursing organization, the Society of Superintendents of Training Schools (eventually the National League for Nursing Education and, then, the National League for Nursing). Robb became the first president of the Nurses Associated Alumnae of the United States and Canada (now the ANA), was a cofounder of the American Journal of Nursing Company, and was one of the founders of the International Council of Nurses. She helped nursing to become an organized profession at the turn of the last century.

Individuals can sometimes bring about social change, eventually accruing a like-minded group behind them. However, social change is also brought about by well-placed collective action.

From the early days of the Code, nurses were seen to have civic responsibilities as well as duties of citizenship, both of which received emphasis. Participatory citizenship by nurses has been a consistent and important thread through the various versions of the Code. By 1960, the Code became explicit with regard to a nurse's duty to attend to legislative matters, individually and collectively.

As a professional person, the nurse's special background enables her to have a greater understanding of the nature of health problems. This understanding poses a particular responsibility to interpret and speak out in regard to legislation affecting health. The resources of the professional association enables the nurse to work with colleagues in assessing current or pending health legislation and its effect upon the community and to determine the stand that should be taken in the interest of the greatest possible good. Sometimes this stand may lead to concerted action with other health groups. At other times, nurses may find it necessary to work alone to support principles which the profession believes will result in the greatest benefits to patient care.[26]

In its interpretive statement for Provision 9, the 2001 Code of Ethics is both more direct and more succinct on the responsibility of the professional association in shaping healthcare policy and legislation, an example of the third function of social ethics. It embraces the emphasis on citizenship responsibilities of previous

Codes, but is more incisive and aggressive about collective/professional association responsibility. It bears restatement:

> Nurses can work individually as citizens or collectively through political action to bring about social change. It is the responsibility of a professional nursing association to speak for nurses collectively in shaping and reshaping health care within our nation, specifically in areas of healthcare policy and legislation that affect accessibility, quality, and the cost of health care. Here the professional association maintains vigilance and takes action to influence legislators, reimbursement agencies, nursing organizations, and other health professions. In these activities, health is understood as being broader than delivery and reimbursement systems, but extending to health-related sociocultural issues such as violation of human rights, homelessness, hunger, violence, and the stigma of illness.

While the new Code does not precisely redefine *health*, it extends the vision of health and of working for the health of all to include both health broadly defined and, more specifically, the social causes of ill health: homelessness, hunger, violence, stigma, and the violation of human rights. A concern for poverty would be intrinsic to these concerns.

Has the Association done this? A look at the ANA government affairs web page is instructive. It has two divisions: Federal Advocacy and State Government Relations. At these web pages, there is access to the ANA legislative and regulatory agenda for the current session of Congress. There are issues analyses, legislative tracking, vote scorecards and information for all members of Congress, legislative updates, federal agency monitoring, a link to the *Federal Register*, a Nurses' Strategic Action Team, and an ANA Political Action Committee. In terms of state legislation regarding health care, the ANA State Relations webpage has links to a host of political resources, a means of identifying one's state and federal legislators, a list of nurse-legislators by state, information in each state's legislation from 1996 to the present, transcripts of ANA testimony before state legislators (and Congress), and more. Over the past two decades, ANA has become exceedingly well organized for influencing the shape of legislation affecting health care, nursing practice, and education. This has been aided by the rise of the Internet that allows greater and more immediate communication with ANA members (and anyone who accesses the website) regarding legislative issues. The ANA has been active in giving testimony before legislators, in communicating with individual legislators, and in bringing the collective concern of nurses to bear upon health legislation. The Association is meeting its duty to be vigilant and to engage with the legislative process. Are the activities of the Association effective in this arena? The duty is to be involved—not necessarily to succeed. ANA is involved on behalf of nursing and nurses. As to whether ANA per se is successful in effecting change, that remains an excellent arena for evaluation research.

Provision 9 of the new Code of Ethics incorporates concerns of earlier Codes for participatory citizenship, for meeting civic responsibilities, for speaking out, both individually and collectively, regarding health and nursing-related legislation. It also encompasses the historic activism of nurses in bringing about social change. However, this provision crystallizes the role of professional associations (not just the ANA) in social ethics on behalf of the profession. In doing so, it addresses the three functions of social ethics. This Code of Ethics, finally, gives greater emphasis to what has historically been a preeminent concern of nursing; the shape of society as it affects health.

Endnotes

1   Gibson, W. 1966. *Elements for a Social Ethics*, p. 215. New York: Macmillan.

2. Fowler, M.D.M. 1972. Nursing and social ethics. In *The Nursing Profession: Turning Points,* N.A. Chaska, ed., pp. 24–30, St. Louis: C.V. Mosby.

3. Perlman C., and L. Olbrechts-Tyteca. 1969. *The New Rhetoric: A Treatise on Argumentation,* p. 51, Notre Dame: Notre Dame University.

4. Ibid.

5. Fowler, 1972. *Nursing,* p. 24–30.

6. National League for Nursing Education. 1917. *Standard Curriculum for Schools of Nursing.* New York: NLNE.

7. Bureau of Registration of Nurses, California State Board of Health. 1916. *Schools of Nursing Requirements and Curriculum,* pp. 7–8, 19–21, 66–67, 83–85, 105–106. Sacramento: State Printing Office.

8. Convention of Training School Alumnae Delegates and Representatives from the American Society of Superintendents of Training Schools for Nurses. 1896. *Proceedings of the Con- vention, 2–4 November 1896,* p. 7. Harrisburg: Harrisburg Publishing.

9. Fowler, M. 2006. Ethics, the profession and society. In *The Teaching of Nursing Ethics: Content and Methods,* Anne Davis, Louise de Raeve, and Verena Tschudin, eds. London: Elsevier.

10. American Nurses Association. 2001. *Code of Ethics for Nurses with Interpretive Statements*, p. 25. Washington, DC: ANA.

11. American Nurses Association website. http://nursingworld.org/ethics/ecode.htm.

12. American Nurses Association. 1964. *Suggested Guidelines for Handling Alleged Violations of the Code for Professional Nurses*. New York: ANA.

13. Ibid, p. 1.

14. American Nurses Association. 2001. Code of Ethics, p. 25.

15. American Nurses Association. 1985. *Code for Nurses with Interpretive Statements*, p. 14, Kansas City, MO: ANA.

16. American Nurses Association. 1976. *Code for Nurses with Interpretive Statements*, pp. 16–17. Kansas City, MO: ANA.

17. American Nurses Association. 1960. *Interpretation of the Statements of the Code for Professional Nurses*, p.13. New York: ANA.

18. American Nurses Association. 1926. A Suggested Code. *American Journal of Nursing* 26(8): 599–601.

19. American Nurses Association. 1940. A Tentative Code. *American Journal of Nursing* 40(9): 978.

20. American Nurses Association. 1950. *The Code for Professional Nurses*. New York: ANA.

21. American Nurses Association. 2001. The Code of Ethics for Nurses, p.25.

22. American Nurses Association. 1940. A Tentative Code, p. 980.

23. American Nurses Association. 1950. The Code for Professional Nurses.

24. American Nurses Association. 2001. Code of Ethics, p. 25.

25. Katz, Esther, ed. 2002. *The Selected Papers of Margaret Sanger, Volume I: The Woman Rebel, 1900–1928*. Chicago: University of Illinois.

26. American Nurses Association. 1960. The Code for Professional Nurses, p. 9.

Guide to the Code of Ethics for Nurses

About the Author

Marsha D.M. Fowler, PhD, MDiv, MS, RN, FAAN, is Senior Fellow and Professor of Ethics, Spirituality, and Faith Integration at Azusa Pacific University. She is a graduate of Kaiser Foundation School of Nursing (diploma), University of California at San Francisco (BS, MS), Fuller Theological Seminary (MDiv), and the University of Southern California (PhD). She has engaged in teaching and research in bioethics and spirituality since 1974. Her research interests are in the history and development of nursing ethics and the Code of Ethics for Nurses, social ethics and professions, suffering, the intersections of spirituality and ethics, and religious ethics in nursing. Dr. Fowler is also a Fellow in the American Academy of Nursing.

Appendix A

Code of Ethics for Nurses with Interpretive Statements

(American Nurses Association, 2001)

Citation note: The content of this appendix (pages 138–169) is a reproduction of the 2001 publication *Code of Ethics for Nurses with Interpretive Statements*, (ISBN: 978-1-55810-176-0), which is in print as a stand-alone publication. The per-page content of each version, however, will differ, due to the different sizes and layout of the two publications. One can cite from or use as a reference either the 2001 primary source or this version. What is important is to ensure that any citation of or reference to *Code of Ethics for Nurses with Interpretive Statements* denotes the 2001 publication and copyright date, not the date of *Guide to the Code of Ethics for Nurses: Interpretation and Application.*

Library of Congress Cataloging-in-Publication Data

Code of ethics for nurses with interpretive statements.
    p. ; cm.
  ISBN 1-55810-176-4
   1. Nursing ethics. I. American Nurses Association.
   [DNLM: 1. Ethics, Nursing. 2. Ethics, Professional. WY 85 C669 2001]
  RT85 .C63 2001
  174'.2–dc21

2001046340

The American Nurses Association (ANA) is a national professional association. ANA's Code of Ethics for Nurses and the accompanying Interpretive Statements reflect the thinking of the nursing profession on various issues and should be reviewed in conjunction with state board of nursing policies and practices. State law, rules, and regulations govern the practice of nursing, while the Code of Ethics guides nurses in the application of their professional skills and personal responsibilities.

Published by Nursesbooks.org
The Publishing Program of ANA
American Nurses Association
8515 Georgia Avenue
Silver Spring, MD 2910-3492
1-800-274-4ANA
http://www.nursesbooks.org/

ANA is the only full-service professional organization representing the nation's 2.9 million Registered Nurses through its 54 constituent member associations. ANA advances the nursing profession by fostering high standards of nursing practice, promoting the economic and general welfare of nurses in the workplace, projecting a positive and realistic view of nursing, and by lobbying the Congress and regulatory agencies on health care issues affecting nurses and the public.

First printing August 2001. Second printing February 2002. Third printing November 2003. Fourth printing December 2004. Fifth printing April 2007.

ISBN-13: 978-1-55810-176-0 CEN21 30M 04/07R
ISBN-10: 1-55810-176-4

Acknowledgments

Members of the Code of Ethics Project Task Force

Barbara Daly, PhD, RN (*Chairperson*)
Elaine Connolly, MS, RN, ANA (*Board of Directors*)
Theresa Drought, PhD, RN
Marsha Fowler, PhD, MDiv, MS, RN, FAAN
Patricia Murphy, PhD, RN, CS, FAAN, ANA (*Board of Directors*)
Linda Olson, PhD, RN
Kathleen Poi, MS, RN, CNAA
Gloria Ramsey, RN, JD
Mary Cipriano Silva, PhD, RN, FAAN
Colleen Scanlon, RN, MS, JD (*Consultant*)
Molly Sullivan, RN
John Twomey, PNP, PhD

ANA Staff

Laurie Badzek, RN, MS, JD, LLM
Director (1998–1999; 2003–present)
Center for Ethics and Human Rights

Gladys White, PhD, RN
Former Director, (2000–2003)

Angela Thompson
Ethics Coordinator (1997–2001)

Contents

Code of Ethics for Nurses

PROVISION 1

The nurse, in all professional relationships, practices with compassion and respect for the inherent dignity, worth and uniqueness of every individual, unrestricted by considerations of social or economic status, personal attributes, or the nature of health problems.

PROVISION 2

The nurse's primary commitment is to the patient, whether an individual, family, group or community.

PROVISION 3

The nurse promotes, advocates for and strives to protect the health, safety and rights of the patient.

PROVISION 4

The nurse is responsible and accountable for individual nursing practice and determines the appropriate delegation of tasks consistent with the nurse's obligation to provide optimum patient care.

PROVISION 5

The nurse owes the same duties to self as to others, including the responsibility to preserve integrity and safety, to maintain competence and to continue personal and professional growth.

PROVISION 6

The nurse participates in establishing, maintaining and improving healthcare environments and conditions of employment conducive to the provision of quality health care and consistent with the values of the profession through individual and collective action.

PROVISION 7

The nurse participates in the advancement of the profession through contributions to practice, education, administration, and knowledge development.

PROVISION 8

The nurse collaborates with other health professionals and the public in promoting community, national, and international efforts to meet health needs.

PROVISION 9

The profession of nursing, as represented by associations and their members, is responsible for articulating nursing values, for maintaining the integrity of the profession and its practice and for shaping social policy.

Preface

Ethics is an integral part of the foundation of nursing. Nursing has a distinguished history of concern for the welfare of the sick, injured, and vulnerable and for social justice. This concern is embodied in the provision of nursing care to individuals and the community. Nursing encompasses the prevention of illness, the alleviation of suffering, and the protection, promotion, and restoration of health in the care of individuals, families, groups, and communities. Nurses act to change those aspects of social structures that detract from health and well-being. Individuals who become nurses are expected not only to adhere to the ideals and moral norms of the profession but also to embrace them as a part of what it means to be a nurse. The ethical tradition of nursing is self-reflective, enduring, and distinctive. A code of ethics makes explicit the primary goals, values, and obligations of the profession.

The Code of Ethics for Nurses serves the following purposes:

- It is a succinct statement of the ethical obligations and duties of every individual who enters the nursing profession.

- It is the profession's nonnegotiable ethical standard.

- It is an expression of nursing's own understanding of its commitment to society.

There are numerous approaches for addressing ethics; these include adopting or subscribing to ethical theories, including humanist, feminist, and social ethics, adhering to ethical principles, and cultivating virtues. The Code of Ethics for Nurses reflects all of these approaches. The words "ethical" and "moral" are used throughout the Code of Ethics. "Ethical" is used to refer to reasons for decisions about how one ought to act, using the above mentioned approaches. In general, the word "moral" overlaps with "ethical" but is more aligned with personal belief and cultural values. Statements that describe activities and attributes of nurses in this Code of Ethics are to be understood as normative or prescriptive statements expressing expectations of ethical behavior.

The Code of Ethics for Nurses uses the term *patient* to refer to recipients of nursing care. The derivation of this word refers to "one who suffers," reflecting a universal aspect of human existence. Nonetheless, it is recognized that nurses also provide services to those seeking health as well as those responding to illness, to students and to staff, in healthcare facilities as well as in communities. Similarly, the term *practice* refers to the actions of the nurse in whatever role the nurse fulfills, including direct patient care provider, educator, administrator, researcher, policy developer, or other. Thus, the values and obligations expressed in this Code of Ethics apply to nurses in all roles and settings.

The Code of Ethics for Nurses is a dynamic document. As nursing and its social context change, changes to the Code of Ethics are also necessary. The Code of Ethics consists of two components: the provisions and the accompanying interpretive statements. There are nine provisions. The first three describe the most fundamental values and commitments of the nurse; the next three address boundaries of duty and loyalty, and the last three address aspects of duties beyond individual patient encounters. For each provision, there are interpretive statements that provide greater specificity for practice and are responsive to the contemporary context of nursing. Consequently, the interpretive statements are subject to more frequent revision than are the provisions. Additional ethical guidance and detail can be found in ANA or constituent member association position statements that address clinical, research, administrative, educational, or public policy issues.

The Code of Ethics for Nurses with Interpretive Statements provides a framework for nurses to use in ethical analysis and decision-making. The Code of Ethics establishes the ethical standard for the profession. It is not negotiable in any setting nor is it subject to revision or amendment except by formal process of the House of Delegates of the ANA. The Code of Ethics for Nurses is a reflection of the proud ethical heritage of nursing, a guide for nurses now and in the future.

Code of Ethics for Nurses with Interpretive Statements

1 The nurse, in all professional relationships, practices with compassion and respect for the inherent dignity, worth, and uniqueness of every individual, unrestricted by considerations of social or economic status, personal attributes, or the nature of health problems

1.1 Respect for human dignity

A fundamental principle that underlies all nursing practice is respect for the inherent worth, dignity, and human rights of every individual. Nurses take into account the needs and values of all persons in all professional relationships.

1.2 Relationships to patients

The need for health care is universal, transcending all individual differences. The nurse establishes relationships and delivers nursing services with respect for human needs and values, and without prejudice. An individual's lifestyle, value system and religious beliefs should be considered in planning health care with and for each patient. Such consideration does not suggest that the nurse necessarily agrees with or condones certain individual choices, but that the nurse respects the patient as a person.

1.3 The nature of health problems

The nurse respects the worth, dignity and rights of all human beings irrespective of the nature of the health problem. The worth of the person is not affected by disease, disability, functional status, or proximity to death. This respect extends to all who require the services of the nurse for the promotion of health, the prevention of illness, the restoration of health, the alleviation of suffering, and the provision of supportive care to those who are dying.

The measures nurses take to care for the patient enable the patient to live with as much physical, emotional, social, and spiritual well-being as possible. Nursing care aims to maximize the values that the patient has treasured in life and extends supportive care to the family and significant others. Nursing care is directed toward meeting the comprehensive needs of patients and their families across the continuum of care. This is particularly vital in the care of patients and their families at the end of life to prevent and relieve the cascade of symptoms and suffering that are commonly associated with dying.

Nurses are leaders and vigilant advocates for the delivery of dignified and humane care. Nurses actively participate in assessing and assuring the responsible and appropriate use of interventions in order to minimize unwarranted or unwanted treatment and patient suffering. The acceptability and importance of carefully considered decisions regarding resuscitation status, withholding and withdraw-ing life-sustaining therapies, forgoing medically provided nutrition and hydration, aggressive pain and symptom management and advance directives are increasingly evident. The nurse should provide interventions to relieve pain and other symptoms in the dying patient even when those interventions entail risks of hastening death. However, nurses may not act with the sole intent of ending a patient's life even though such action may be motivated by compassion, respect for patient autonomy and quality of life considerations. Nurses have invaluable experience, knowledge, and insight into care at the end of life and should be actively involved in related research, education, practice, and policy development.

1.4 The right to self-determination

Respect for human dignity requires the recognition of specific patient rights, particu-larly, the right of self-determination. Self-determination, also known as autonomy, is the philosophical basis for informed consent in health care. Patients have the moral and legal right to determine what will be done with their own person; to be given accurate, complete, and understandable information in a manner that facilitates an informed judgment; to be assisted with weighing the benefits, burdens, and available options in their treatment, including the choice of no treatment; to accept, refuse, or terminate treatment without deceit, undue influence, duress, coercion, or penalty; and to be given necessary support throughout the decision-making and treatment process. Such support would include the opportunity to make decisions with family and significant others and the provision of advice and support from knowledgeable nurses and other health professionals. Patients should be involved in planning their own health care to the extent they are able and choose to participate.

Each nurse has an obligation to be knowledgeable about the moral and legal rights of all patients to self-determination. The nurse preserves, protects, and supports those interests by assessing the patient's comprehension of both the information presented and the implications of decisions. In situations in which the patient lacks the capacity to make a decision, a designated surrogate decision-maker should be consulted. The role of the surrogate is to make decisions as the patient would, based upon the patient's previously expressed wishes and known values. In the absence of a designated surrogate decision-maker, decisions should be made in the best interests of the patient, considering the patient's personal values to the extent that they are known. The nurse supports patient self-determination by participating in discussions with surrogates, providing guidance and referral to other resources as necessary, and identifying and addressing problems in the decision-making process. Support of autonomy in the broadest sense also includes recognition that people of some cultures place less weight on individualism and choose to defer to family or community values in decision-making. Respect not just for the specific decision but also for the patient's method of decision-making is consistent with the principle of autonomy.

Individuals are interdependent members of the community. The nurse recognizes that there are situations in which the right to individual self-determination may be outweighed or limited by the rights, health and welfare of others, particularly in relation to public health considerations. Nonetheless, limitation of individual rights must always be considered a serious deviation from the standard of care, justified only when there are no less restrictive means available to preserve the rights of others and the demands of justice.

1.5 Relationships with colleagues and others

The principle of respect for persons extends to all individuals with whom the nurse interacts. The nurse maintains compassionate and caring relationships with colleagues and others with a commitment to the fair treatment of individuals, to integrity-preserving compromise, and to resolving conflict. Nurses function in many roles, including direct care provider, administrator, educator, researcher, and consultant. In each of these roles, the nurse treats colleagues, employees, assistants, and students with respect and compassion. This standard of conduct precludes any and all prejudicial actions, any form of harassment or threatening behavior, or disregard for the effect of one's actions on others. The nurse values the distinctive contribution of individuals or groups, and collaborates to meet the shared goal of providing quality health services.

2 The nurse's primary commitment is to the patient, whether an individual, family, group, or community.

2.1 Primacy of the patient's interests

The nurse's primary commitment is to the recipient of nursing and healthcare services—the patient—whether the recipient is an individual, a family, a group, or a community. Nursing holds a fundamental commitment to the uniqueness of the individual patient; therefore, any plan of care must reflect that uniqueness. The nurse strives to provide patients with opportunities to participate in planning care, assures that patients find the plans acceptable and supports the implementation of the plan. Addressing patient interests requires recognition of the patient's place in the family or other networks of relationship. When the patient's wishes are in conflict with others, the nurse seeks to help resolve the conflict. Where conflict persists, the nurse's commitment remains to the identified patient.

2.2 Conflict of interest for nurses

Nurses are frequently put in situations of conflict arising from competing loyalties in the workplace, including situations of conflicting expectations from patients, families, physicians, colleagues, and in many cases, healthcare organizations and health plans. Nurses must examine the conflicts arising between their own personal and professional values, the values and interests of others who are also responsible for patient care and healthcare decisions, as well as those of patients. Nurses strive to resolve such conflicts in ways that ensure patient safety, guard the patient's best interests and preserve the professional integrity of the nurse.

Situations created by changes in healthcare financing and delivery systems, such as incentive systems to decrease spending, pose new possibilities of conflict between economic self-interest and professional integrity. The use of bonuses, sanctions, and incentives tied to financial targets are examples of features of healthcare systems that may present such conflict. Conflicts of interest may arise in any domain of nursing activity including clinical practice, administration, education, or research. Advanced practice nurses who bill directly for services and nursing executives with budgetary responsibilities must be especially cognizant of the potential for conflicts of interest. Nurses should disclose to all relevant parties (e.g., patients, employers, colleagues) any perceived or actual conflict of interest and in some situations should withdraw from further participation. Nurses in all roles must seek to ensure that employment arrangements are just and fair and do not create an unreasonable conflict between patient care and direct personal gain.

2.3 Collaboration

Collaboration is not just cooperation, but it is the concerted effort of individuals and groups to attain a shared goal. In health care, that goal is to address the health needs of the patient and the public. The complexity of healthcare delivery systems requires a multi-disciplinary approach to the delivery of services that has the strong support and active participation of all the health professions. Within this context, nursing's unique contribution, scope of practice, and relationship with other health professions needs to be clearly articulated, represented and preserved. By its very nature, collaboration requires mutual trust, recognition, and respect among the healthcare team, shared decision-making about patient care, and open dialogue among all parties who have an interest in and a concern for health outcomes. Nurses should work to assure that the relevant parties are involved and have a voice in decision-making about patient care issues. Nurses should see that the questions that need to be addressed are asked and that the information needed for informed decision-making is available and provided. Nurses should actively promote the collaborative multi-disciplinary planning required to ensure the availability and accessibility of quality health services to all persons who have needs for health care.

Intra-professional collaboration within nursing is fundamental to effectively addressing the health needs of patients and the public. Nurses engaged in non-clinical roles, such as administration or research, while not providing direct care, nonetheless are collaborating in the provision of care through their influence and direction of those who do. Effective nursing care is accomplished through the interdependence of nurses in differing roles—those who teach the needed skills, set standards, manage the environment of care, or expand the boundaries of knowledge used by the profession. In this sense, nurses in all roles share a responsibility for the outcomes of nursing care.

2.4 Professional boundaries

When acting within one's role as a professional, the nurse recognizes and maintains boundaries that establish appropriate limits to relationships. While the nature of nursing work has an inherently personal component, nurse-patient relationships and nurse-colleague relationships have, as their foundation, the purpose of preventing illness, alleviating suffering, and protecting, promoting, and restoring the health of patients. In this way, nurse-patient and nurse-colleague relationships differ from those that are purely personal and unstructured, such as friendship. The intimate nature of nursing care, the involvement of nurses is important and sometimes highly stressful life events, and the mutual dependence of colleagues working in close concert all present the potential for blurring of limits to professional relationships. Maintaining authenticity and expressing oneself as an individual, while remaining within the bounds established by the purpose of the relationship can be especially difficult in prolonged or long-term relationships. In all encounters, nurses are responsible for retaining their professional boundaries. When those professional boundaries are jeopardized, the nurse should seek assistance from peers or supervisors or take appropriate steps to remove her/himself from the situation.

3 The nurse promotes, advocates for, and strives to protect the health, safety, and rights of the patient.

3.1 Privacy

The nurse safeguards the patient's right to privacy. The need for health care does not justify unwanted intrusion into the patient's life. The nurse advocates for an environment that provides for sufficient physical privacy, including privacy for discussions of a personal nature and policies and practices that protect the confidentiality of information.

3.2 Confidentiality

Associated with the right to privacy, the nurse has a duty to maintain confidentiality of all patient information. The patient's well-being could be jeopardized and the fundamental trust between patient and nurse destroyed by unnecessary access to data or by the inappropriate disclosure of identifiable patient information. The rights, well-being, and safety of the individual patient should be the primary factors in arriving at any professional judgment concerning the disposition of confidential information received from or about the patient, whether oral, written or electronic. The standard of nursing practice and the nurse's responsibility to provide quality care require that relevant data be shared with those members of the healthcare team who have a need to know. Only information pertinent to a patient's treatment and welfare is disclosed, and only to those directly involved with the patient's care. Duties of confidentiality, however, are not absolute and may need to be modified in order to protect the patient, other innocent parties and in circumstances of mandatory disclosure for public health reasons.

Information used for purposes of peer review, third-party payments, and other quality improvement or risk management mechanisms may be disclosed only under defined policies, mandates, or protocols. These written guidelines must assure that the rights, well-being, and safety of the patient are protected. In general, only that information directly relevant to a task or specific responsibility should be disclosed. When using electronic communications, special effort should be made to maintain data security.

3.3 Protection of participants in research

Stemming from the right to self-determination, each individual has the right to choose whether or not to participate in research. It is imperative that the patient or legally authorized surrogate receive sufficient information that is material to an informed decision, to comprehend that information, and to know how to discontinue participation in research without penalty. Necessary information to achieve an adequately informed consent includes the nature of participation, potential harms and benefits, and available alternatives to taking part in the research. Additionally, the patient should be informed of how the data will be protected. The patient has the right to refuse to participate in research or to withdraw at any time without fear of adverse consequences or reprisal.

Research should be conducted and directed only by qualified persons. Prior to implementation, all research should be approved by a qualified review board to ensure patient protection and the ethical integrity of the research. Nurses should be cognizant of the special concerns raised by research involving vulnerable groups, including children, prisoners, students, the elderly, and the poor. The nurse who participates in research in any capacity should be fully informed about both the subject's and the nurse's rights and obligations in the particular research study and in research in general. Nurses have the duty to question and, if necessary, to report and to refuse to participate in research they deem morally objectionable.

3.4 Standards and review mechanisms

Nursing is responsible and accountable for assuring that only those individuals who have demonstrated the knowledge, skill, practice experiences, commitment, and integrity essential to professional practice are allowed to enter into and continue to practice within the profession. Nurse educators have a responsibility to ensure that basic competencies are achieved and to promote a commitment to professional practice prior to entry of an individual into practice. Nurse administrators are responsible for assuring that the knowledge and skills of each nurse in the workplace are assessed prior to the assignment of responsibilities requiring preparation beyond basic academic programs.

The nurse has a responsibility to implement and maintain standards of professional nursing practice. The nurse should participate in planning, establishing, implementing, and evaluating review mechanisms designed to safeguard patients and nurses, such as peer review processes or committees, credentialing processes, quality improvement initiatives, and ethics committees. Nurse administrators must ensure that nurses have access to and inclusion on institutional ethics committees. Nurses must bring forward difficult issues related to patient care and/ or institutional constraints upon ethical practice for discussion and review. The nurse acts to promote inclusion of appropriate others in all deliberations related to patient care.

Nurses should also be active participants in the development of policies and review mechanisms designed to promote patient safety, reduce the likelihood of errors, and address both environmental system factors and human factors that present increased risk to patients. In addition, when errors do occur, nurses are expected to follow institutional guidelines in reporting errors committed or observed to the appropriate supervisory personnel and for assuring responsible disclosure of errors to patients. Under no circumstances should the nurse participate in, or condone through silence, either an attempt to hide an error or a punitive response that serves only to fix blame rather than correct the conditions that led to the error.

3.5 Acting on questionable practice

The nurse's primary commitment is to the health, well-being, and safety of the patient across the life span and in all settings in which healthcare needs are addressed. As an advocate for the patient, the nurse must be alert to and take appropriate action regarding any instances of incompetent, unethical, illegal, or impaired practice by any member of the healthcare team or the healthcare system or any action on the part of others that places the rights or best interests of the patient in jeopardy. To function effectively in this role, nurses must be knowledgeable about the Code of Ethics, standards of practice of the profession, relevant federal, state and local laws and regulations, and the employing organization's policies and procedures.

When the nurse is aware of inappropriate or questionable practice in the provision or denial of health care, concern should be expressed to the person carrying out the questionable practice. Attention should be called to the possible detrimental affect upon the patient's well-being or best interests as well as the integrity of nursing practice. When factors in the healthcare delivery system or healthcare organization threaten the welfare of the patient, similar action should be directed to the responsible administrator. If indicated, the problem should be reported to an appropriate higher authority within the institution or agency, or to an appropriate external authority.

There should be established processes for reporting and handling incompetent, unethical, illegal, or impaired practice within the employment setting so that such reporting can go through official channels, thereby reducing the risk of reprisal against the reporting nurse. All nurses have a responsibility to assist those who identify potentially questionable practice. State nurses associations should be prepared to provide assistance and support in the development and evaluation of such processes and reporting procedures.When incompetent, unethical, illegal, or impaired practice is not corrected within the employment setting and continues to jeopardize patient well-being and safety, the problem should be reported to other appropriate authorities such as practice committees of the pertinent professional organizations, the legally constituted bodies concerned with licensing of specific categories of health workers and professional practitioners, or the regulatory agencies concerned with evaluating standards or practice. Some situations may warrant the concern and involvement of all such groups. Accurate reporting and factual documentation, and not merely opinion, undergird all such responsible actions. When a nurse chooses to engage in the act of responsible reporting about situations that are perceived as unethical, incompetent, illegal, or impaired, the professional organization has a responsibility to provide the nurse with support and assistance and to protect the practice of those nurses who choose to voice their concerns. Reporting unethical, illegal, incompetent, or impaired practices, even when done appropriately, may present substantial risks to the nurse; nevertheless, such risks do not eliminate the obligation to address serious threats to patient safety.

3.6 Addressing impaired practice

Nurses must be vigilant to protect the patient, the public and the profession from potential harm when a colleague's practice, in any setting, appears to be impaired. The nurse extends compassion and caring to colleagues who are in recovery from illness or when illness interferes with job performance. In a situation where a nurse suspects another's practice may be impaired, the nurse's duty is to take action designed both to protect patients and to assure that the impaired individual receives assistance in regaining optimal function. Such action should usually begin with consulting supervisory personnel and may also include confronting the individual in a supportive manner and with the assistance of others or helping the individual to access appropriate resources. Nurses are encouraged to follow guidelines outlined by the profession and policies of the employing organization to assist colleagues whose job performance may be adversely affected by mental or physical illness or by personal circumstances. Nurses in all roles should advocate for colleagues whose job performance may be impaired to ensure that they receive appropriate assistance, treatment and access to fair institutional and legal processes. This includes supporting the return to practice of the individual who has sought assistance and is ready to resume professional duties.

If impaired practice poses a threat or danger to self or others, regardless of whether the individual has sought help, the nurse must take action to report the individual to persons authorized to address the problem. Nurses who advocate for others whose job performance creates a risk for harm should be protected from negative consequences. Advocacy may be a difficult process and the nurse is advised to follow workplace policies. If workplace policies do not exist or are inappropriate—that is, they deny the nurse in question access to due legal process or demand resignation—the reporting nurse may obtain guidance from the professional association, state peer assistance programs, employee assistance program or a similar resource.

4 The nurse is responsible and accountable for individual nursing practice and determines the appropriate delegation of tasks consistent with the nurse's obligation to provide optimum patient care

4.1 Acceptance of accountability and responsibility

Individual registered nurses bear primary responsibility for the nursing care that their patients receive and are individually accountable for their own practice. Nursing practice includes direct care activities, acts of delegation, and other responsibilities such as teaching, research, and administration. In each instance, the nurse retains accountability and responsibility for the quality of practice and for conformity with standards of care.

Nurses are faced with decisions in the context of the increased complexity and changing patterns in the delivery of health care. As the scope of nursing practice changes, the nurse must exercise judgment in accepting responsibilities, seeking consultation, and assigning activities to others who carry out nursing care. For example, some advanced practice nurses have the authority to issue prescription and treatment orders to be carried out by other nurses. These acts are not acts of delegation. Both the advanced practice nurse issuing the order and the nurse

Guide to the Code of Ethics for Nurses

accepting the order are responsible for the judgments made and accountable for the actions taken.

4.2 Accountability for nursing judgment and action

Accountability means to be answerable to oneself and others for one's own actions. In order to be accountable, nurses act under a code of ethical conduct that is grounded in the moral principles of fidelity and respect for the dignity, worth, and self-determination of patients. Nurses are accountable for judgments made and actions taken in the course of nursing practice, irrespective of healthcare organizations' policies or providers' directives.

4.3 Responsibility for nursing judgment and action

Responsibility refers to the specific accountability or liability associated with the performance of duties of a particular role. Nurses accept or reject specific role demands based upon their education, knowledge, competence, and extent of experience. Nurses in administration, education, and research also have obligations to the recipients of nursing care. Although nurses in administration, education, and research have relationships with patients that are less direct, in assuming the responsibilities of a particular role, they share responsibility for the care provided by those whom they supervise and instruct. The nurse must not engage in practices prohibited by law or delegate activities to others that are prohibited by the practice acts of other healthcare providers.

Individual nurses are responsible for assessing their own competence. When the needs of the patient are beyond the qualifications and competencies of the nurse, consultation and collaboration must be sought from qualified nurses, other health professionals, or other appropriate sources. Educational resources should be sought by nurses and provided by institutions to maintain and advance the competence of nurses. Nurse educators act in collaboration with their students to assess the learning needs of the student, the effectiveness of the teaching program, the identification and utilization of appropriate resources, and the support needed for the learning process.

4.4 Delegation of nursing activities

Since the nurse is accountable for the quality of nursing care given to patients, nurses are accountable for the assignment of nursing responsibilities to other nurses and the delegation of nursing care activities to other healthcare workers. While delegation and assignment are used here in a generic moral sense, it is understood that individual states may have a particular legal definition of these terms.

The nurse must make reasonable efforts to assess individual competence when assigning selected components of nursing care to other healthcare workers. This assessment involves evaluating the knowledge, skills, and experience of the individual to whom the care is assigned, the complexity of the assigned tasks, and the health status of the patient. The nurse is also responsible for monitoring the activities of these individuals and evaluating the quality of the care provided. Nurses may not delegate responsibilities such as assessment and evaluation; they may delegate tasks. The nurse must not knowingly assign or delegate to any member of the nursing team a task for which that person is not prepared or qualified. Employer policies or directives do not relieve the nurse of responsibility for making judgments about the delegation and assignment of nursing care tasks.

Nurses functioning in management or administrative roles have a particular responsibility to provide an environment that supports and facilitates appropriate assignment and delegation. This includes providing appropriate orientation to staff, assisting less experienced nurses in developing necessary skills and competencies, and establishing policies and procedures that protect both the patient and nurse from the inappropriate assignment or delegation of nursing responsibilities, activities, or tasks.

Nurses functioning in educator or preceptor roles may have less direct relationships with patients. However, through assignment of nursing care activities to learners they share responsibility and accountability for the care provided. It is imperative that the knowledge and skills of the learner be sufficient to provide the assigned nursing care and that appropriate supervision be provided to protect both the patient and the learner.

5 The nurse owes the same duties to self as to others, including the responsibility to preserve integrity and safety, to maintain competence, and to continue personal and professional growth.

5.1 Moral self-respect

Moral respect accords moral worth and dignity to all human beings irrespective of their personal attributes or life situation. Such respect extends to oneself as well; the same duties that we owe to others we owe to ourselves. Self-regarding duties refer to a realm of duties that primarily concern oneself and include professional growth and maintenance of competence, preservation of wholeness of character, and personal integrity.

5.2 Professional growth and maintenance of competence

Though it has consequences for others, maintenance of competence and ongoing professional growth involves the control of one's own conduct in a way that is primarily self-regarding. Competence affects one's self-respect, self-esteem, professional status, and the meaningfulness of work. In all nursing roles, evaluation of one's own performance, coupled with peer review, is a means by which nursing practice can be held to the highest standards. Each nurse is responsible for participating in the development of criteria for evaluation of practice and for using those criteria in peer and self-assessment.

Continual professional growth, particularly in knowledge and skill, requires a commitment to lifelong learning. Such learning includes, but is not limited to, continuing education, networking with professional colleagues, self-study, professional reading, certification, and seeking advanced degrees. Nurses are required to have knowledge relevant to the current scope and standards of nursing practice, changing issues, concerns, controversies, and ethics. Where the care required is outside the competencies of the individual nurse, consultation should be sought or the patient should be referred to others for appropriate care.

5.3 Wholeness of character

Nurses have both personal and professional identities that are neither entirely separate, nor entirely merged, but are integrated. In the process of becoming a professional, the nurse embraces the values of the profession, integrating them with personal values. Duties to self involve an authentic expression of one's own moral point-of-view in practice. Sound ethical decision-making requires the respectful and open exchange of views between and among all individuals with relevant interests. In a community of moral discourse, no one person's view should automatically take precedence over that of another. Thus the nurse has a responsibility to express moral perspectives, even when they differ from those of others, and even when they might not prevail.

This wholeness of character encompasses relationships with patients. In situations where the patient requests a personal opinion from the nurse, the nurse is generally free to express an informed personal opinion as long as this preserves the voluntariness of the patient and maintains appropriate professional and moral boundaries. It is essential to be aware of the potential for undue influence attached to the nurse's professional role. Assisting patients to clarify their own values in reaching informed decisions may be helpful in avoiding unintended persuasion. In situations where nurses' responsibilities include care for those whose personal attributes, condition, lifestyle or situation is stigmatized by the community and are personally unacceptable, the nurse still renders respectful and skilled care.

5.4 Preservation of integrity

Integrity is an aspect of wholeness of character and is primarily a self-concern of the individual nurse. An economically constrained healthcare environment presents the nurse with particularly troubling threats to integrity. Threats to integrity may include a request to deceive a patient, to withhold information, or to falsify records, as well as verbal abuse from patients or coworkers. Threats to integrity also may include an expectation that the nurse will act in a way that is inconsistent with the values or ethics of the profession, or more specifically a request that is in direct violation of the Code of Ethics. Nurses have a duty to remain consistent with both their personal and professional values and to accept compromise only to the degree that it remains an integrity-preserving compromise. An integrity-preserving compromise does not jeopardize the dignity or well-being of the nurse or others. Integrity-preserving compromise can be difficult to achieve, but is more likely to be accomplished in situations where there is an open forum for moral discourse and an atmosphere of mutual respect and regard.

Where nurses are placed in situations of compromise that exceed acceptable moral limits or involve violations of the moral standards of the profession, whether in direct patient care or in any other forms of nursing practice, they may express their conscientious objection to participation. Where a particular treatment, intervention, activity, or practice is morally objectionable to the nurse, whether intrinsically so or because it is inappropriate for the specific patient, or where it may jeopardize both patients and nursing practice, the nurse is justified in refusing to participate on moral grounds. Such grounds exclude personal preference, prejudice, convenience, or arbitrariness. Conscientious objection may not insulate the nurse against formal or informal penalty. The nurse who decides not to take part on the grounds of conscientious objection must communicate this decision in appropriate ways. Whenever possible, such a refusal should be made known in advance and in time for alternate arrangements to be made for patient care. The nurse is obliged to provide for the patient's safety, to avoid patient abandonment, and to withdraw only when assured that alternative sources of nursing care are available to the patient.

Where patterns of institutional behavior or professional practice compromise the integrity of all its nurses, nurses should express their concern or conscientious objection collectively to the appropriate body or committee. In addition, they should express their concern, resist, and seek to bring about a change in those persistent activities or expectations in the practice setting that are morally objectionable to nurses and jeopardize either patient or nurse well-being.

6 The nurse participates in establishing, maintaining, and improving healthcare environments and conditions of employment conducive to the provision of quality health care and consistent with the values of the profession through individual and collective action.

6.1 Influence of the environment on moral virtues and values

Virtues are habits of character that predispose persons to meet their moral obligations; that is, to do what is right. Excellences are habits of character that predispose a person to do a particular job or task well. Virtues such as wisdom, honesty, and courage are habits or attributes of the morally good person. Excellences such as compassion, patience, and skill are habits of character of the morally good nurse. For the nurse, virtues and excellences are those habits that affirm and promote the values of human dignity, well-being, respect, health, independence, and other values central to nursing. Both virtues and excellences, as aspects of moral character, can be either nurtured by the environment in which the nurse practices or they can be diminished or thwarted. All nurses have a responsibility to create, maintain, and contribute to environments that support the growth of virtues and excellences and enable nurses to fulfill their ethical obligations.

6.2 Influence of the environment on ethical obligations

All nurses, regardless of role, have a responsibility to create, maintain, and contribute to environments of practice that support nurses in fulfilling their ethical obligations. Environments of practice include observable features, such as working conditions, and written policies and procedures setting out expectations for nurses, as well as less tangible characteristics such as informal peer norms. Organizational structures, role descriptions, health and safety initiatives, grievance mechanisms, ethics committees, compensation systems, and disciplinary procedures all contribute to environments that can either present barriers or foster ethical practice and professional fulfillment. Environments in which employees are provided fair hearing of grievances, are supported in practicing according to standards of care, and are justly treated allow for the realization of the values of the profession and are consistent with sound nursing practice.

6.3 Responsibility for the healthcare environment

The nurse is responsible for contributing to a moral environment that encourages respectful interactions with colleagues, support of peers, and identification of issues that need to be addressed. Nurse administrators have a particular responsibility to assure that employees are treated fairly and that nurses are involved in decisions related to their practice and working conditions. Acquiescing and accepting unsafe or inappropriate practices, even if the individual does not participate in the specific practice, is equivalent to condoning unsafe practice. Nurses should not remain employed in facilities that routinely violate patient rights or require nurses to severely and repeatedly compromise standards of practice or personal morality.

As with concerns about patient care, nurses should address concerns about the healthcare environment through appropriate channels. Organizational changes are difficult to accomplish and may require persistent efforts over time. Toward this end, nurses may participate in collective action such as collective bargaining or workplace advocacy, preferably through a professional association such as the state nurses association, in order to address the terms and conditions of employment. Agreements reached through such action must be consistent with the profession's standards of practice, the state law regulating practice and the Code of Ethics for Nursing. Conditions of employment must contribute to the moral environment, the provision of quality patient care and professional satisfaction for nurses.

The professional association also serves as an advocate for the nurse by seeking to secure just compensation and humane working conditions for nurses. To accomplish this, the professional association may engage in collective bargaining on behalf of nurses. While seeking to assure just economic and general welfare for nurses, collective bargaining, nonetheless, seeks to keep the interests of both nurses and patients in balance.

7 The nurse participates in the advancement of the profession through contributions to practice, education, administration, and knowledge development.

7.1 Advancing the profession through active involvement in nursing and in healthcare policy

Nurses should advance their profession by contributing in some way to the leadership, activities, and the viability of their professional organizations. Nurses can also advance the profession by serving in leadership or mentorship roles or on committees within their places of employment. Nurses who are self-employed can advance the profession by serving as role models for professional integrity. Nurses can also advance the profession through participation in civic activities related to health care or through local, state, national, or international initiatives. Nurse educators have a specific responsibility to enhance students' commitment to professional and civic values. Nurse administrators have a responsibility to foster an employment environment that facilitates nurses' ethical integrity and professionalism, and nurse researchers are responsible for active contribution to the body of knowledge supporting and advancing nursing practice.

7.2 Advancing the profession by developing, maintaining, and implementing professional standards in clinical, administrative, and educational practice

Standards and guidelines reflect the practice of nursing grounded in ethical commitments and a body of knowledge. Professional standards and guidelines for nurses must be developed by nurses and reflect nursing's responsibility to society. It is the responsibility of nurses to identify their own scope of practice as permitted by professional practice standards and guidelines, by state and federal laws, by relevant societal values, and by the Code of Ethics.

The nurse as administrator or manager must establish, maintain, and promote conditions of employment that enable nurses within that organization or community setting to practice in accord with accepted standards of nursing practice and provide a nursing and healthcare work environment that meets the standards and guidelines of nursing practice. Professional autonomy and self regulation in the control of conditions of practice are necessary for implementing nursing standards and guidelines and assuring quality care for those whom nursing serves.

The nurse educator is responsible for promoting and maintaining optimum standards of both nursing education and of nursing practice in any settings where planned learning activities occur. Nurse educators must also ensure that only those students who possess the knowledge, skills, and competencies that are essential to nursing graduate from their nursing programs.

7.3 Advancing the profession through knowledge development, dissemination, and application to practice

The nursing profession should engage in scholarly inquiry to identify, evaluate, refine, and expand the body of knowledge that forms the foundation of its discipline and practice. In addition, nursing knowledge is derived from the sciences and from the humanities. Ongoing scholarly activities are essential to fulfilling a profession's obligations to society. All nurses working alone or in collaboration with others can participate in the advancement of the profession through the development, evaluation, dissemination, and application of knowledge in practice. However, an organizational climate and infrastructure conducive to scholarly inquiry must be valued and implemented for this to occur.

8 The nurse collaborates with other health professionals and the public in promoting community, national, and international efforts to meet health needs.

8.1 Health needs and concerns

The nursing profession is committed to promoting the health, welfare, and safety of all people. The nurse has a responsibility to be aware not only of specific health needs of individual patients but also of broader health concerns such as world hunger, environmental pollution, lack of access to health care, violation of human rights, and inequitable distribution of nursing and healthcare resources. The availability and accessibility of high quality health services to all people require both interdisciplinary planning and collaborative partnerships among health professionals and others at the community, national, and international levels.

8.2 Responsibilities to the public

Nurses, individually and collectively, have a responsibility to be knowledgeable about the health status of the community and existing threats to health and safety. Through support of and participation in community organizations and groups, the nurse assists in efforts to educate the public, facilitates informed choice, identifies conditions and circumstances that contribute to illness, injury and disease, fosters healthy life styles, and participates in institutional and legislative efforts to promote health and meet national health objectives. In addition, the nurse supports initiatives to address barriers to health, such as poverty, homelessness, unsafe living conditions, abuse and violence, and lack of access to health services.

The nurse also recognizes that health care is provided to culturally diverse populations in this country and in all parts of the world. In providing care, the nurse should avoid imposition of the nurse's own cultural values upon others. The nurse should affirm human dignity and show respect for the values and practices associated with different cultures and use approaches to care that reflect awareness and sensitivity.

9 The profession of nursing, as represented by associations and their members, is responsible for articulating nursing values, for maintaining the integrity of the profession and its practice, and for shaping social policy.

9.1 Assertion of values

It is the responsibility of a professional association to communicate and affirm the values of the profession to its members. It is essential that the professional organization encourages discourse that supports critical self-reflection and evaluation within the profession. The organization also communicates to the public the values that nursing considers central to social change that will enhance health.

9.2 The profession carries out its collective responsibility through professional associations

The nursing profession continues to develop ways to clarify nursing's accountability to society. The contract between the profession and society is made explicit through such mechanisms as (a) The Code of Ethics for Nurses, (b) the standards of nursing practice, (c) the ongoing development of nursing knowledge derived from nursing theory, scholarship, and research in order to guide nursing actions, (d) educational requirements for practice, (e) certification, and (f) mechanisms for evaluating the effectiveness of professional nursing actions.

9.3 Intraprofessional integrity

A professional association is responsible for expressing the values and ethics of the profession and also for encouraging the professional organization and its members to function in accord with those values and ethics. Thus, one of its fundamental responsibilities is to promote awareness of and adherence to the Code of Ethics and to critique the activities and ends of the professional association itself. Values and ethics influence the power structures of the association in guiding, correcting, and directing its activities. Legitimate concerns for the self-interest of the association and the profession are balanced by a commitment to the social goods that are sought. Through critical self-reflection and self-evaluation, associations must foster change within themselves, seeking to move the professional community toward its stated ideals.

9.4 Social reform

Nurses can work individually as citizens or collectively through political action to bring about social change. It is the responsibility of a professional nursing association to speak for nurses collectively in shaping and reshaping health care within our nation, specifically in areas of healthcare policy and legislation that affect accessibility, quality, and the cost of health care. Here, the professional association maintains vigilance and takes action to influence legislators, reimbursement agencies, nursing organizations, and other health professions. In these activities, health is understood as being broader than delivery and reimbursement systems, but extending to health-related sociocultural issues such as violation of human rights, homelessness, hunger, violence, and the stigma of illness.

Afterword

The development of the *Code of Ethics for Nurses with Interpretive Statements* is a benchmark for both the American Nurses Association and for the profession of nursing as a whole. The evolution of the Code dates from 1893 when the "Nightingale Pledge" was adopted, and from 1926 and 1940 when tentative Codes were suggested but not formally ratified. This is the first time in the last 25 years that the entire Code has been revised and the second time in the last 50 years that an entirely new document has been produced. This Code is the result of five years of work on the part of the Code of Ethics Project Task Force, an advisory board, state liaisons, and ANA staff. It is the culmination of more than ten field reviews of drafts that were circulated in hard copy and made available online, incorporating comments from hundreds of nurses across the United States and abroad.

The ethical tradition that has been manifest in every iteration of the Code is self-reflective, enduring, and distinctive. The ethical standard established by the Code of Ethics is nonnegotiable. This means that the Code supports the nurse in a steadfast way across various settings and in a variety of nursing roles. This Code of Ethics is for all nurses and is particularly useful at the beginning of the 21st century because it: reiterates the fundamental values and commitments of the nurse (provisions 1–3); identifies the boundaries of duty and loyalty (provisions 4–6); and describes the duties of the nurse that extend beyond individual patient encounters (provisions 7–9). The achievement of a true global awareness about the human condition and the needs for health care is one of the most important moral challenges of the 21st century and this Code beckons nurses toward such an awareness.

The Code of Ethics is the promise that nurses are doing their best to provide care for their patients and their communities, supporting each other in the process so that all nurses can fulfill their ethical and professional obligations. This *Code of Ethics for Nurses with Interpretive Statements* is an important tool that can be used now as leverage to a better future for nurses, patients, and health care.

Timeline:
The Evolution of Nursing's Code of Ethics

Whatever the version of the Code, it has always been fundamentally concerned with the principles of doing no harm, of benefitting others, of loyalty, and of truthfulness. As well, the Code has been concerned with social justice and, in later versions, with the changing context of health care as well as the autonomy of the patient and the nurse.

1893 The "Nightingale Pledge, " patterned after medicine's Hippocratic Oath, is understood as the first nursing code of ethics.

1896 The Nurses' Associated Alumnae of the United States and Canada (later to become the American Nurses Association), whose first purpose was to establish and maintain a code of ethics.

1926 "A Suggested Code" is provisionally adopted and published in the American Journal of Nursing (AJN) but is never formally adopted.

1940 "A Tentative Code" is published in AJN, but also is never formally adopted.

1950 The Code for Professional Nurses, in the form of 17 provisions that are a substantive revision of the "Tentative Code" of 1940, is unanimously accepted by the ANA House of Delegates.

1956 The Code for Professional Nurses is amended.

1960 The Code for Professional Nurses is revised.

1968 The Code for Professional Nurses is substantively revised, condensing the 17 provisions of the 1960 Code into 10 provisions.

1976 The *Code for Nurses with Interpretive Statements*, a modification of the provisions and interpretive statements, is published as 11 provisions.

1985 The *Code for Nurses with Interpretive Statements* retains the provisions of the 1976 version and includes revised interpretive statements.

2001 The *Code for Nurses with Interpretive Statements* is accepted by the ANA House of Delegates.

Index

Guide to the Code of Ethics for Nurses